Recovering from Depression, Anxiety, and Psychosis

My Journey Through Mental Illness

Formerly titled *Cry Depression...*

BY BARBARA ALTMAN

ISBN: 1477499016

ISBN 13: 9781477499016

Author's Disclaimer

You must know that everything I say in this book is based upon my experience with battling depression, psychosis, and anxiety disorder. There are many people who would not embrace the type of treatment I've pursued and who would disagree with an alternative approach to mental illness. If you pursue the treatments I've outlined at the end of the book without the supervision of a licensed medical doctor, you do so at your own risk. The book producer, author, and bookstores present this information for educational purposes only. I'm not making an attempt to prescribe any medical treatment, as only a licensed medical doctor can do so. I'm a musician, not an MD.

While the protocols outlined at the end of the book worked for me, there is no guarantee it will work for others. The last psychotic event occurred at the age of nineteen, long before I looked into alternative methods. Therefore, the system of health care I've used was not curative, but was implemented in the hopes of fine-tuning my health.

Barbara Altman

Dedication

This book is dedicated with abundant love to all those who have enriched my life:

Mom (whose love nurtured and sustained me through many frustrations)

Dad (who was one of my best teachers)

My Grandmother and Grandfather Tritz (who served as surrogate parents)

My Grandmother and Grandfather Schneider (who loved and supported me)

All of my wonderful piano and guitar students

All of the wonderful elderly residents in the nursing homes I serve

My Aunt Girlie McGhee, Aunt Alma Tritz, Aunt Gina Ryan

My Aunt Annie Altman Franke

My Uncle Carl Franke

My Uncle Edmund and my Uncle Russell McGhee

My brother, Jack Altman, and my four nephews: John, David, Mark, and Jeffrey Altman

My friend Rosemary Banayat Bennett

All those involved in helping me heal my body, mind, and spirit

In loving memory of my father, Edward John Altman
b. August 20, 1899; d. October 30, 1976.

In loving memory of my mother, Laura Altman
b. August 31, 1909; d. February 17, 1995.

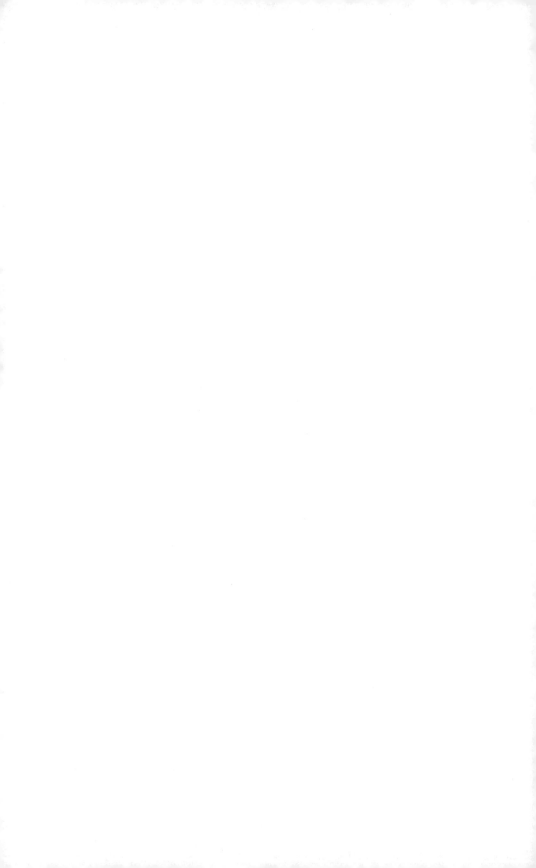

Contents

Author's Disclaimer iii

Dedication v

Preface xiii

Acknowledgements xv

Introduction xvii

Section One, Part One

Chapter 1   Father's Day: 2004, Age 61. 3

Chapter 2   The Principal's Office: 1960, Age 16 5

Chapter 3   Driving to Kansas: 1986, Age 42 9

Chapter 4   The Large Ant: 1949, Age 6 13

Chapter 5   Cleaning Up Larned, Kansas: 1986, Age 42. 15

Chapter 6   State Mental Hospital: 1959, Age 16 17

Chapter 7   The Weekly Card Game: 1953, Age 10 19

Chapter 8   Classes at Larned: 1986, Age 42. 23

Chapter 9   The Piano Lesson: 1951, Age 8 25

Chapter 10   In the Swim: 1972, Age 28 27

Chapter 11   Sugar, Sweet or Sour: 1958, Age 15. 29

Chapter 12   In Jail: 1986, Age 42. 31

Chapter 13   "The Three Faces of Eve:" 1958, Age 15. 35

Chapter 14   Grandmothers, Mother, and Daughter:
              1955 – 1958, Ages 12 – 15 37

Chapter 15   Teachers and Counselors at
              Larned: 1986, Age 42. 39

Chapter 16   The Lunchroom: 1958, Age 15 41

Chapter 17   Leaving Larned: 1986, Age 42 43

Chapter 18   The Fontbonne Years: 1961 – 1965,
              Ages 17 – 21 45

Chapter 19   Two Trips to Hell: 1961, Age 18 49

Chapter 20   The St. Louis Institute of Music:
              1969 – 1985, Ages 26 – 42 53

Chapter 21   European Adventures: 1970; Age 27 57

Chapter 22   Confrontation: 1973, Age 30 61

Chapter 23   Bethesda-Dilworth: 1986, Age 42 63

Chapter 24   Music Therapy with the Elderly:
              1998, Age 55 67

Chapter 25   My Father's Final Years: 1972 – 1976,
              Ages 29 – 33 71

Chapter 26   My Mother's Final Years:
              1992 – 1995, Ages 49 – 52 75

Chapter 27   Trying to Heal My Body: 1987 – 1989,
              Ages 43 – 45 81

Section One, Part Two

Chapter 28   Therapy – Creating the Will to
              Live: 1989, Age 46 87

Chapter 29   Painting New Pictures: 1989, Age 46 91

Chapter 30   Group Therapy: 1998, Age 55 95

Chapter 31   Observe and Emulate: 2002, Age 59 97

Chapter 32   Songs and Social Skills: June 2005, Age 62 101

Chapter 33   Trial and Error: 2004, Age 61 103

Chapter 34   Mastering Fears: 2008, Age 65 107

The Feathered Parade 111

Section Two

Introduction 115

Chapter 1   Descriptions of a Few Mental Health
Disorders 119

Chapter 2   Traditional Medical Treatments 127

Chapter 3   Counseling 129

Chapter 4   Complementary (Alternative) Therapies. 131

Author's Epilogue

Appendix A   Recommended Readings 139

Appendix B   Living the Joy-Filled Life: Affirmations. 141

Appendix C   Improving My Health. 145

You can contact Barbara Altman through her website
http://www.depressiontorecovery.com.

Preface

Praise and many thanks go to that wonderful carpenter from Bethlehem, who has been the light of my life.

I grew up in a fear-based environment. Family members worried about small events, but offered little protection in dangerous situations. Triple locks graced every door. Crossing the street in a safe area brought warnings, and I heard "be careful" more often than I care to remember. They painted the image of a dangerous world. We had both good and bad times, and we shared a lot of love, coupled with a bushel of dysfunction.

This book isn't just a story about the struggles involved with mental illness. It isn't only about a family's survival through the trauma of alcoholism or the anguish of anxiety disorder. And it's not about blaming my father. It's about God's goodness shining forth in those who devote their lives to helping the mentally ill; it's about my transformation from victim to survivor and from mental illness to health. With the help of my family, several counselors, support groups, and physicians, I've assumed a position of health, strength, and passion.

It takes a village to help the mentally ill.

Acknowledgements

I want to extend my thanks to Renee Wallace for her many trips to my house to repair my computer woes.

To Ray Fezzi, I extend my hand of gratitude for his professional aid when I returned from my music therapy internship. He guided me through a difficult job adjustment at Bethesda-Dillworth Nursing Home.

To Lanette Kellie, I say thank you for firing me from my music therapy internship at Larned State Hospital in Larned, Kansas. Was that ever a wake-up call!

To my wonderful team of doctors, I say, "God bless you." You've offered me another chance at having a sound, stable mind.

Marigene and Larry DaRusha have given me the gift of their wonderful teachings and spiritual support at the Center for Spiritual Living in Maryland Heights, Missouri.

I thank Melanie DePorter, Bonnie Sievers, Anna Thomas, and Lois Duncan for their feedback, and Linda Senn for her patient and comprehensive service as my book coach. I also thank Eileen P. Duggan and Vera Glick for copyediting the manuscript.

I couldn't have accomplished this task without the assistance of Louise and Kenneth Portwine, who patiently edited and typed the first manuscript from two hundred hand-written pages.

To Burt and Dana St. John, I say thank you for your editorial efforts and for helping me establish the format of this book.

Special gratitude is extended to Caroline Penberthy for the eighteen years of counsel and friendship. Caroline held my hand through my transition from anorexia to health and helped me fan the flames of the will to live.

To Patricia Antle, I offer my fondest appreciation for her support during the years after my father's death. Patricia helped me to dim the flames of resentment I held toward both my parents.

Introduction

My credentials, education, and work experience revolve around music education and music therapy. I'm not a traditional or an alternative healing expert. I'm an adult child of an alcoholic, a survivor of major depressive episodes, psychosis, and chronic anxiety. I've used a combination of diet, lifestyle, and integrative healing approaches, which have enabled me to build a satisfying and successful life. By the age of nineteen, all major psychotic episodes had ceased years before I began my aggressive treatment modalities. I did, however, continue to have problems with concentration, focus, depression, and anxiety. My eclectic regimen has been designed to manage these symptoms.

Many of the incidents recounted in this book occurred more than fifty years ago. Things were said and events happened that were significant to my development. While I can't guarantee one hundred percent dialogue accuracy, my story is based on truth. Others may remember things differently.

I changed some names in order to maintain the anonymity of the patients at Larned State Mental Hospital and of the residents of three local nursing homes where I provide music therapy.

I live in the present, striving to build a life I love, and I share my story in the hopes that it might encourage anyone who's had to deal with depression, psychosis, or anxiety.

It's been deeply painful and therapeutic for me to reflect upon my past and to relive and reframe it with despair and hope, sadness and humor, and promise and faith.

So my dear readers, grab hold of your spectacles. You're in for a ride full of drama, sadness, and happy prospects.

SECTION 1
Part One

The Girl without a Voice

*Would my father ever see the pain in
my eyes or the ache in my soul?*

CHAPTER ONE

Father's Day: 2004, Age 61

For me, that Father's Day was a day of profound grief. Even though his small yellowing photo looked much like the others on the Center for Spiritual Living's simple wooden alter, the memory of his drinking and the abuse made me weep.

From the picture, the man standing beside his dapple gray horse and Pevely Dairy milk wagon looked normal. But Dad had inherited alcoholic behavior, a crippling self-image, and a lack of life purpose from his father. Memories of an unhappy childhood haunted him.

His dark mantra was: "We're all nothing more than miserable ants crawling on the earth. God can crush us at will."

He felt the pain of not living up to his potential as a husband, father, and provider. "Barbara despises me because I'm a milkman and a member of the rank and file. Some of her friends come from rich families, and she resents me because we're poor." He brainwashed my mother with this and she passed it on to me.

But I loved being the child of blue-collar workers and the granddaughter of a janitor. The hearty blue-collar work ethic appealed to my childlike nature.

My heart swelled with pride whenever he showed me pictures of his horse and milk wagon. An employee of various dairies from the twenties through the fifties, his duties required him to deliver milk products door-to-door throughout the St. Louis area.

Our problems were exacerbated by his drinking, screaming, temper tantrums, and verbal abuse. We didn't experience boundaries, trust, or warmth. My parents didn't invest any interest in my education except to make sure I got to school. Dad drank every night of the week, and Mother had to work two or three evenings a week as a checker at Schnucks grocery store. Many evenings were spent alone in an ocean of tears.

While walking home from school, I'd wonder if he'd be there. An empty garage always produced a broken heart.

How I yearned for his presence!

Would my father ever see the pain in my eyes or the ache in my soul? Would he acknowledge the existence of his second child? Would he finally step up to the plate and soothe his daughter's pain?

His addiction blinded him to his family's suffering.

CHAPTER TWO

The Principal's Office: 1960, Age 16

Why did the principal want to see me? She didn't call students into her office for anything but serious reasons. What did I do? Is she upset because I didn't turn in my history assignment? Am I being confronted for not paying attention in class? Did I rub one of my teachers the wrong way? I sat in her waiting room with those questions in mind when she opened the door and asked me to come in.

Her room felt cold. I closed the door to the sounds of rambunctious teenaged girls chattering down the hall and entered the inner sanctum of "Mother God."

Even in her traditional black nun's garb, she appeared tall, thin, and domineering, with large hands that commanded attention.

Three lonely books on her desk and a stark wall clock defined the mood of her office. Time seemed endless as she began to speak those life-changing words to me.

"Barbara, we're concerned about the problems you're having in the classroom." Her towering presence was thoroughly intimidating. "I've checked your IQ scores, and your grades aren't in line with your abilities. I'm getting reports that you're not concentrating in any of your classes. In my opinion, you're on the verge of developing full-blown

schizophrenia. If you don't see a psychiatrist immediately, you'll end up in a mental institution for the rest of your life."

I sobbed. I knew she was right, but everything in me screamed No! I'm going to get a music scholarship, go to college, and become an independent music teacher. Wasting my life in a psychiatric hospital doesn't fit the plan! My vision included living successfully in society.

I'd set a firm intention. I was going to make it!

I didn't tell her about my experience with anxiety, depression, and psychotic events. The first two were obvious. But I'd hoped to conceal the last reality, never letting anyone know about my frequent auditory hallucinations. Disclosure of that would've gotten me a quick ticket to the nearest mental institution.

She proceeded to set up an appointment with my mother. The meeting between those strong-willed women was shrill, as I could hear all too well in the waiting room.

"Barbara's heading toward a total mental breakdown. She's schizophrenic and needs help now."

"She's not mentally ill. I'll never believe that. Things at home aren't ideal. It's her father . . ."

They continued yelling for about forty-five minutes. The principal finally won her point and set up an appointment for my parents and me with Monsignor Behrmann, the director of special education for the Archdiocese of St. Louis.

My experience with him was the first of frequent, positive encounters with members of the mental health community. I arrived at his office feeling anxious and depressed. Was he going to institutionalize me? Would I have to give up my dream of going to college? Would he treat me like some kind of misfit because I was having all these problems? Would he brand me "mentally ill"?

The soft blue carpet hinted at the kindness therein. The wealth of mental health literature in his bookcase testified to his knowledge and caring.

A gray-haired, muscular man in his fifties, he proved to be warm and compassionate.

"Barbara, I'm going to give you a battery of tests, one of which will determine your IQ. We'll start with a series of questions," he began, settling into his worn desk chair.

"If a tree grows to be eight inches tall in a year, twelve inches in the second year, and eighteen inches in the third year, how tall will it be in the fourth year?"

I smoothed down the pleats in my uniform skirt, pondered for a moment, and came up with the correct answer. "Twenty-seven," I said triumphantly.

"You're right!" He smiled like a proud uncle.

"Where will you end up if you start walking in a northerly direction, followed by walking east, then south, and west?"

I missed that one. I said I would end up south of where I started.

I was questioned for about another forty-five minutes and was told not to doubt my mental capabilities. As the session wore on, I became more and more at ease with his approach and less fearful of the session's outcome.

The decision was made to set up an appointment with a psychiatrist who would, hopefully, be able to shed some light on my predicament. I was to visit both the doctor and Monsignor separately once a month.

Before I left, Monsignor had me kneel on the floor to receive his blessing. He gently placed his hands on my head and prayed God's favor on me.

I left feeling warm and loved.

One week later, my parents and I entered the downtown office of Dr. Robert Lamm, a trim, clean-shaven, Filipino, who wasn't always easy for me to understand. He recommended I be given an EEG (electroencephalogram), which records brain activity.

Feeling a bit queasy, I left Mom and Dad in the waiting area and walked into the small, spare exam room. The "electric chair" sitting in the corner, and the dime-sized window, gave the room a sterile feel.

Nurse Ratchet, a.k.a. "Cuckoo's Nest," skewered me with about two dozen blood-sucking needles, which she jabbed into my tender scalp. I was truly nailed in place!

Dr. Lamm had been told about my problems with temporary blackouts and concentration. I was both shocked and proud to hear the diagnosis of petit mal epilepsy. I was given Phenobarbital to prevent further seizures (blackouts).

During the ensuing months, I had to see him on a regular basis with a report of my symptoms. The medication stopped the seizures, but did nothing for the unremitting brain fog.

Would I be lost in that fog for the rest of my life? Would no doctor be able to help me? Would no one understand my pain? The despair was crushing.

This was my "cross" to bear, my identity with redemptive suffering. I'd have to wait more than forty years to experience relief.

CHAPTER THREE

Driving to Kansas: 1986, Age 42

My long-awaited departure date, June 10, 1986, had finally arrived. After two years of preliminary study in Music Therapy at Maryville, I took off on the eleven-hour journey to Larned State Mental Hospital in western Kansas. At age forty-two, I was about to begin my internship there, an experience that was to be monitored by several members of the hospital staff.

I'd packed clothes, reference books, and enough cash to pay for gasoline and food to get me there. My saddest and flattest facial expressions and my quiet nature came along for the ride. I left St. Louis intending to exorcise the demons plaguing me since the age of six.

Suitcases in hand, I stood in my mother's living room and bade farewell to the old Steinway grand piano, the music stand, and the dear pictures of musicians on the wall. Sadly, I left all the symbols of my love for music behind.

Adieu, old friends.

The counterpoint to the sadness was the abrupt good-bye to my family. No kisses and no hugs.

Adventure lay ahead. The drive west to Kansas City on Highway 70 was filled with lush green hillsides and fields of wildflowers along the fertile Missouri River valley. The car radio played the classical music so dear to me since childhood. I thought about the life I was leaving behind, not realizing this kind of thinking might invite the same kind of life into my future.

Skydiving couldn't have been more terrifying than weaving through a multitude of cars over tricky overpasses with their tangles of highway signs. Then Missouri's pastoral scenery changed to the boring Kansas flatlands and oil rigs.

Larned couldn't be too far off, I thought. Instead, I drove another six hours. I was ready to give up when I finally saw the Larned sign.

After another twenty minutes, I arrived in town and pulled into the lone filling station, where I waited for my supervisor, Lanette Kellie.

That last scrubby mile to the hospital was the longest.

I'd expected a campus of two or three buildings. But Larned was a sprawling campus of seventy-five acres with housing for both lifelong and short-term residents, medium and maximum security prisons, a library, and an activities building. All the hospital structures were widely separated by land. The complex existed to serve residents with challenges ranging from age-related senility, schizophrenia, drug addiction, schizoaffective and bipolar disorders, and depression, to roughly sixty at-risk young people from dysfunctional families. The grassy lawns and plantings on the spacious hospital grounds were kept restrained by a team of gardeners. In addition, there was a block of twelve, small, white cottages that housed interns and employees.

My fellow intern, Coreen, dubbed her accommodations "The Little House on the Prairie," while I named mine "The Ritz-Carlton." I decided to apply some elbow grease to my little house. Armed with Clorox and Lysol, I began to scour my grimy quarters.

After hours of work, my cottage felt like a fresh start. And I had my place in good order and pleasant enough to consider the possibility of enjoying my temporary stay there.

It was time to begin my journey of dealing with people who were mentally ill just like me. The story of my life points to that reality. I was middle-aged and had been living with a compromised mind since childhood.

CHAPTER FOUR

The Large Ant: 1949, Age 6

I was six years old, and I wanted a Brown Cow from the milkman.

"Mommy, can I have a nickel for some ice cream? Please, please, please?"

I stood on the cracked, once-white linoleum floor in the kitchen. The room spoke of the everyday life of a blue-collar family. The sink was stained and worn with many years' use as were the cabinets below it. The plain cotton curtains at the window over that sink hung limp and motionless in the heat of the summer morning.

My mother left her ironing board long enough to fish a nickel out of the jar on top of the refrigerator and handed it to me absent-mindedly. I ran out the back door, no doubt letting it slam, across the concrete patio, and into the front yard.

The milkman's coming! The bell on his truck rang with a loud ding, ding, ding. Hurry! Run! Run, Barbara, run! Sweat poured down my face and I drooled with anticipation. I was out of breath from running and so excited. The truck ground to a slow, squeaky halt.

The driver smiled kindly. "Good morning, Barbara. What do you want today?"

"I want a Brown Cow," I said, dancing a little jig on the sidewalk.

He pulled the sweet treat off the truck, and I immediately began to devour that yummy ice cream as he drove on down the pot-holed street toward the railroad tracks.

Completely focused on my ice cream, I turned toward the house. There, in front of me on the concrete, I saw an enormous, terrifying ant nearly as tall as me, with huge feelers reaching out to attack. Gulping down my terror, I charged up to it and stamped my foot, shouting, "Go away. Go away!"

Then I turned away, hoping with every fiber of my little body that it would leave on its own. When I look again, will it be gone or will it be as big as the house? I didn't stay long enough to find out. Dropping my prized Brown Cow on the pavement, I bolted into the backyard and up the steps. In the kitchen I found my mother, still at the ironing board, sliding the hot iron back and forth over my father's blue work shirts.

Panting, I cried, "Mommy, I saw a big bug, a huge ant." No response. Silently, I yelled, "Stop ironing! Look at me!"

Finally my mother looked up from her task, tucking a stray curl behind her ear as she looked at me. Tick tock, like the beating of a clock, her movements were predictable and familiar, but they were not comforting to her frightened child. I stretched out my six-year-old arms to show the size of the monster. I was screaming inside.

Looking irritated, she waved her hand at me. "You probably just saw a water bug, Barbara."

"It's too big to be a water bug." The pitch of my voice reached a new intensity. I extended my arms out as far as they'd go and tried to describe the horrific experience. I didn't know the word "hallucination." She didn't either. No doubt she figured I had an overactive imagination. Struggling against what I'd seen, my mind simply went blank.

She turned her back on me and went back to her ironing. I stopped talking. I stopped screaming. I became mute, thinking, "It was a big ant. It was. It was."

My arms dropped to my sides.

I was angry. I was scared. I was silent.

CHAPTER FIVE

Cleaning Up Larned, Kansas: 1986, Age 42

The job of cleaning my little house at the hospital in Kansas was completed in five hours. Free to enjoy the rest of the day, I went next door to meet Coreen, my fellow intern. At twenty-three, she was younger, shorter, and rounder than me, with curly brown hair and a well-honed intelligence. She and her family were in the process of unpacking, so we simply introduced ourselves and then parted company, knowing we would be working together the next day.

They provided interns with a detailed six-month calendar. Upon completion, we'd be equipped to deal with schizophrenics, the elderly senile, mentally retarded, at-risk youths, and those with drug addiction problems.

On Monday morning, our supervisor, Lanette, met with us in her sparse mini-conference room, and gave us instructions on hospital rules, social do's and don'ts, writing patient reports, and an hour's worth of information.

Staring anxiously at Lanette, I forced myself to concentrate so I could remember everything. *Damn! Would my mind never work like a well-oiled machine?* It all seemed overwhelming. Although failure wasn't an option, anxiety paralyzed my thinking. Mercifully, the room's uncluttered atmosphere had a calming effect on me. The desk clock finally chimed the end of the interview. Both of us were scheduled for a weekly review of our performance, especially professional demeanor and personal interactions.

The first week went smoothly. It was well within my comfort level, as the main tasks were passive observation, writing, and documentation, which have always come easily to me. However, I did feel apprehensive about interacting with both patients and staff.

My persistent mantra was: "There but for the grace of God go I." I had mentally thumbed my nose at the patients. I'd had the brains to beat the system, and they didn't. I was harboring one of the most common prejudices among the mentally ill, namely, "I'm not as sick as you are." While in fact, I was.

My problems began the second week when we were to move beyond observation to patient interaction. I had well-outlined plans for my patient sessions. But when it came time to lead them in an activity, I withered inside. My behavior annoyed both staff and residents, and I began to feel like an intruder. A person with schizophrenia may not show the signs of normal emotion, perhaps may speak in a monotonous voice, have diminished facial expressions, and appear extremely apathetic. This is also known as blunted affect.

"Barbara, we want you to let your hair down," Lanette said. "You don't show any enthusiasm with the staff or patients. We'd like you to at least maintain eye contact. You constantly look lost." When Lanette said that, she had a lively look on her face as though she was modeling that interactive style to me.

Lost. How I hated that word even though that's exactly how I felt. Lanette gave me two weeks to shape up or ship out. How could I escape from my thirty-year paralysis in fourteen days? The answer to that would evolve over the next twenty years.

CHAPTER SIX

State Mental Hospital: 1959, Age 16

My mother and her sister, Gina, had just returned from visiting Gina's husband, Pat, a resident at Farmington State Mental Hospital since 1938. He had hallucinations, fits of violence, and almost a total loss of cognition and bodily function, all the result of syphilis, a little fact that he failed to mention when he and Gina got married! He either chose not to get a penicillin shot or simply didn't get around to it, leaving the disease to ultimately destroy his brain.

The long drive in the steamy St. Louis afternoon didn't begin to explain the haggard, horrified look on her face. "Mom, what's wrong? You look like you're in shock." Gina had simply crumpled into the closest chair, overwhelmed with misery.

"Barbara, I've never seen anything like that ever! Patients were running around naked and walking in their own poop and pee. We're never going back! Neither one of us can take it." Mother stood before me, still stunned by the experience. I'd never seen her look so out of control. Words came fitfully through bouts of weeping. It was a stressful day for all three of us, but especially for her and her sister.

Struck mute, I could only hug and try to comfort her the best way I knew how. I was an immature adolescent, but I consoled her with my heart and my arms.

"I'm sorry that you and Aunt Gina had to see that."

"I refuse to go back. Gina will have a nervous breakdown if she sees him again."

"I don't think you should go back either, Mom." My voice was unusually resolute.

I was already symptomatic. I will never go there either. I won't do that to myself or my family. It seemed no one had noticed my problems. I had enough minimal mental health to "pass," which enabled me to pretend nothing was wrong.

My secret sank into the deepest part of my soul.

CHAPTER SEVEN

The Weekly Card Game: 1953, Age 10

The picture is still vivid for me. We'd gathered at my grandparents' house in Webster Groves for the weekly men's Pinochle game. The kitchen was alive with the sweet aromas of my grandmother's weekly baking. Every Saturday she baked enough fragrant yeast stollens and sugar-sprinkled doughnuts for the following week. The delicious, homey treats were in the oven, being warmed for the family. It was a time for bonding and fun.

The four men sat at the sturdy, wooden, kitchen table in their ritual formation that hadn't changed in twenty years. My grandfather sat at the head. My father, still in his work clothes, was directly opposite him. Quiet Uncle Edmund was at his left, while patient Uncle Bud sat to his right. Thump! Bang! Hands smacked the table.

"Why didn't you play your ace? We coulda had that trick!"

"Shit, I thought that ace was played!"

These comments usually came from my father, who was known to have a temper.

"Don't you know what you're doing?"

Tempers rose, temples throbbed, and veins popped in the heat of competition.

"Cut it out! It's only a game," commented my grandfather.

"Pass the beer." Only my father and grandfather helped themselves this time.

Uncle Edmund puffed a cigar. Aunt Gina walked through with a can of air freshener. *"Good Lord, Edmund! It stinks in here!"*

Male energy ruled that part of the room.

"Mum," said Grandpa, *"muster us up some of those coffeecakes.*

Get it yourself, Pup, she thought, as she turned to fetch them.

While Mum and Pup continued their customary sparring, the men went on a Pinochle rampage, and I was having the time of my young life.

"Oh, Uncle Bud, you have one, two, three, four hairs on the top of your head." I loved standing over Uncle Bud and giving him grief about his thinning hairline.

I then proceeded to count the hairs on the back of his head. He responded patiently to my teasing as only my sweet uncle could do. I eventually tired of playing, and he gave me subtle hints that he wanted to return to Pinochle. I moved around the table to the continued sounds of my father's loud voice. I ignored him and talked with my grandfather and Uncle Edmund.

Suddenly, I felt something icy. *What's going on? Or, rather, what's Aunt doing now?* Regina Carolina Bernadette Tritz, a.k.a. Gina, had put one very cold ice cube down my back. She's the one who put one raw egg on someone's plate every Easter and who'd been known to initiate mashed potato fights at our backyard picnics.

I ran around trying to lose the cube, laughing with my whole body. Knowing one great spiritual truth – what goes around comes around. I grabbed an ice cube from the freezer and sent it down her back. She screamed louder than I had. My grandmother told us to pipe down and stop the shenanigans. We did simmer down.

Now it was my brother's turn. I constantly teased him about his *"mature age"* because he was eleven years older than me and already one very independent young man.

At ten, I stood in awe of my older brother. At the age of twenty-one, he'd already married and was the new father of adorable baby John. In years to come, three more darling little boys, David, Mark, and Jeffrey, were to join the family.

All of this familial giddiness excited my childlike sensibilities, and laughter bubbled out of every pore.

When I needed to regain my composure, I would connect with my beloved mother. That day, as usual, Laura Otillia Tritz Altman, the feisty family storyteller, was holding forth on the creaky front porch with one of her long tales. We all sat mesmerized as she talked about her latest conversation with a friend.

"And I told her . . . I know her like a book! She couldn't have done all of that! . . . I said . . . She said . . . They said . . ."

Most of the story came from her imagination. Not that she was lying. She just liked to expand on reality. From the second word forward, we could take what she said with a grain of salt.

My Aunt Girlie (Alvina) became totally immersed in the yarn. "Laura, you do know how to talk."

It was always good to be on Girlie's side. If she didn't like you, you were beyond help. If she did, she adored you. Fortunately, I was one of the latter.

So I snuggled into her lap as my mother droned on, enjoying the nurturing contact. My favorite Aunt Girlie and Uncle Bud provided me with the only completely secure family connection.

My mother's twin, Aunt Alma, suggested we have a blender milkshake. In the kitchen, I watched her mix milk and chocolate ice cream, and serve it with a dozen or more home-made doughnuts, and fresh apple stollens with white icing drizzled on top.

My grandmother looked at the wooden wall clock and announced, "It's 9:30, time for all good soldiers to hit the hay." My parents had left a little earlier, right before milkshake time.

Cards were put away for another week. Everyone left. It was time for me to go home.

I skipped next door to my house. Then it happened. One minute I was a happy child. Seconds later, I was dying.

I ran into our kitchen, looked past my mother, and saw my father clutching both sides of the doorjamb. Howling and moaning an agonized guttural sound, he swayed back and forth, totally out of control.

I began screaming inside and outside.

"What's wrong with Dad? What's wrong with him?" I froze. Is he about to drop dead in front of me? Mother stared at him in weary

21

sadness, barely seeing me. My father's and my screaming reached a new intensity, mixing in a jagged cacophony of terror and illness.

"Mommy, do something, get a doctor!" I looked at the telephone and wondered why she wasn't calling the hospital. "Call the doctor, he's dying, he's dying!"

I continued to cry unheard screams.

I reached up with my small arms, hoping she'd pick me up and comfort me. Instead, she pushed me behind her in an effort to block him from my view. I clung to her skirt, trying to find my own comfort.

I felt so abandoned, so lost.

Her eyes filled with tears and loneliness; my mother tried to reassure me. "He just found a job at Quality Dairy as a milk driver, and he stopped for a few drinks to celebrate. He drank more at the card game, and he couldn't stop."

"If we're celebrating, why are we all looking so sad?" Shaking all over, I felt an icy chill in my body.

"It's getting late, Barbara," she said. "It's time for you to go to bed."

My mother and I were slipping into denial.

What had just happened to my life?

I felt lost.

I then stopped talking.

I became silent.

My voice had been stolen.

CHAPTER EIGHT

Classes at Larned: 1986, Age 42

I was a forty-two year old music therapy intern, and the horticulture class at Larned continued. Clay pots passed through eight pairs of hands. Peaceful butterflies flitted over our workspace. Patients talked, issues got resolved, and laughter abounded while plants were shared and admired.

Two of the young women, Jane and Sally, suffered from the deep-seated insecurities that often come from living in a dysfunctional family, especially where alcoholism plays a part. But they manifested their problems differently. Sally, a tall, thin twenty-two year old, dressed conservatively, wore a zoned-out look, and acted angry and bitter. Jane was also brunette and about the same age, but carried a few extra pounds on her medium-short frame, and seemed jittery and anxious, often slouching as if to make herself appear smaller. But it was she who opened the conversation.

"Sally, I love your funky hair. Orange is so you," Jane ventured, eyeing Sally's new look.

"I figured you'd think I crossed the line." Sally, who generally had a smart aleck response, seemed to have felt flattered, even sneaking a sideways glance at her friend.

"Of course you have. You always do." Jane's tone softened at the relatively easy conversation.

Six other voices joined in all at once, chattering non-stop throughout the whole gardening class. Talk, laugh, and learn. This was part of their therapy.

As Jane continued to talk about her father, I listened intently.

"It must've been difficult for you to have lived in that situation." Marie, the kindly, maternal instructor, changed the subject as she settled herself onto the wobbly wooden chair beside Jane.

"It was. I've had a hard time with his drinking." Jane looked off into the distance, seeing painful scenes from her past.

"You don't seem to be as nervous as you were when you got here. I think you're making progress." Marie had an old-fashioned way of nodding when she spoke, as though to confirm her statements.

"Thank you."

"We'll keep right on encouraging you to build a life independent of his problems. It just takes a little time to realize that you truly are separate from him and can grow in whatever ways you choose."

The same kind of sympathy, understanding, and support that Jane was receiving would have helped me enormously. However, I did have one healthy outlet. Music and piano were my therapy. Those eight-eight keys comforted me in the middle of my pain and trauma. Beethoven, Chopin, and Mozart became my role models; my music teachers, my mentors. And whenever possible, I'd steal a few minutes to play the piano in the main activity room.

My mother gave me purpose when she signed me up for piano lessons so many years ago.

CHAPTER NINE

The Piano Lesson: 1951, Age 8

Glory day had arrived. For the last six months, my mother had been encouraging me to ask the nuns at my school about piano lessons. I kept putting it off because I really wanted dance and baton instructions. My mother said they were too expensive.

The piano teacher at school had a full schedule, so my mother called Mrs. Lemcke, whose family had music in their genes for several generations. Her husband, Hans, used to play with John Phillip Sousa and led the Webster Groves High School band for at least thirty years. What a treat the community had when he conducted the Memorial Field band concerts every summer!

Thursday afternoons at three-thirty found me at Mrs. Lemcke's studio. For the first lessons, my mother walked me the few blocks from Our Holy Redeemer grade school to the Lemcke home.

My teacher escorted us through the living room of her white, stucco home into the tiny music studio, which housed a small, well-worn spinet. The metronome would have to wait until I actually learned to play.

She sat to my right on a solid oak chair and placed my first piano book, John Thompson's "Teaching Little Fingers How to Play," on the music stand. My mother, seated squarely on the straight-backed chair in the back of the room, silently offered her moral support.

"Barbara, look at the music. The note with a line going through it is called middle C. Place your thumb on it. What do you think the note above it is?" Her grandmotherly appearance felt reassuring.

"D!" I said triumphantly.

"You're right!" She was very effusive with her compliments.

A few minutes later, I played my first song!

For the first time in my life, I felt so proud of me.

"She has talent. She doesn't stumble around like most of them do," Mrs. Lemcke said.

I felt so proud of me!

I sensed my mother's smile before I saw it.

Twelve words and that smile opened my mind and my heart. Two average women in a simple music studio gave me my life. God bless both of them.

Baton and dance lessons flew out the window.

The music bug bit.

CHAPTER TEN

In the Swim: 1972, Age 28

The enormous pool at Larned, with its sharp odor of chlorine and echoes of splashing, reminded me of my own aquatic challenge fifteen years earlier.

I was now twenty-eight years old and determined to finally conquer my fear of deep water. After a six-month struggle, I learned how to swim the width of the Webster YMCA pool, which was an Olympic feat for me! Terrified of the deep, I practiced swimming across the shallow end, which annoyed the lap swimmers.

"Barbara, you're making progress. Keep up the good work." My athletic, sometimes impatient swim instructor shouted her encouragement. All of my instructors urged me on to greater accomplishments.

"I'm trying. I'm determined to swim in the deep water."

At twenty-eight, I was more than old enough to do this.

My way of desensitizing myself has often been through a sequence of tiny goals, and this was a prime example. With my fingers clutching the edge of the pool, I inched my way into the deep, struggling against panic all the way. Week by week I would move a little further down towards the deep end.

One evening, my instructor got frustrated with my miniscule progress and tried for twenty minutes to physically pry my fingers away from the side. Tears ran down my cheeks. Quaking with fear and stiff from holding on, I finally let loose.

She didn't understand the nature of anxiety disorder, that pathological curse of struggle and fear.

I didn't either. Why did God make me like this? How I hated myself and the sorrow plaguing my soul! My body wouldn't cooperate. Weird. That word applied to me. After all, I only wanted one thing: to be able to jump in and swim effortlessly. Was that asking too much?

Sometime after the prying incident, my instructor threw up her hands and yelled, "Barbara, why don't you just let go and swim a lap? I know you can do it." Petrified with fear my hands simply refused to move any more.

"I don't know why I feel like this. I can't explain it." This seemed to temporarily placate her, but it didn't satisfy me. Why did I have to work so hard? Anxiety dimmed the accomplishment of my dreams both in and out of the pool. I felt frustrated with such slow, agonizing progress.

Racing against the next panic attack, I next used a kickboard and rubber fins to speed my progress to the deep end. Success was at hand!

At last, I no longer interrupted the lap swimmers, and I was back in the good graces of everyone. After three months of accomplishing small goals, I negotiated one complete lap.

On and on I fought the fear, hurt, and rage. Oh, how I hated this hopeless life of mine, so filled with despair.

Finally, glory day arrived, and the entire staff came out to give me my Guppy pin. Twelve months of trial and error went into floating and swimming one complete lap. I couldn't do this on anyone else's timetable. It had to be mine. I felt the pride and encouragement offered by the staff. What a scene!

I'd won the battle. But the war still raged.

CHAPTER ELEVEN

Sugar, Sweet or Sour: 1958, Age 15

In 1986, Larned residents would go to the canteen and purchase small items and sugary snacks. I had to abstain because as I'd learned twenty-eight years earlier, I couldn't eat sugar in any quantity.

I was fourteen years old in 1958, and I'd just completed my sophomore year in high school. Those first two years had been difficult, especially socially. Although to provide some perspective, there were islands of happiness even in my worst years.

At the age of fifteen, I met my dear friend Rosemary Banayat at the St. Louis Institute for Music, where we both were enrolled in weekly, Saturday piano lessons. For the next few years, we hung out at the neighborhood Steak 'n' Shake, roller skated, and visited back and forth at each others' homes, developing a normal, healthy friendship that we still enjoy long distance between Arizona and St. Louis.

But those times were the exception. And people who suffer from mental illnesses instantly sink back into deep distress as soon as they wave good-bye.

I spent the rest of my days alone. My parents both worked full time, and my brother was married and gone. Between my overall feelings of inadequacy about myself, life, and in response to my father's drinking and verbal abuse, I spent much of the summer feeding my sugar addiction. I'd eat ice cream for breakfast, candy bars between meals, graham crackers and peanut butter for lunch, more candy bars between lunch and dinner, with a nutritious evening meal served under my mother's wise supervision.

By August my brain was in a deep fog. Even reading the newspaper was difficult. I couldn't concentrate. Fortunately, I regained the ability to focus when school started.

I thought I could do the same thing the following summer. But by then, my reliance on sugar had increased in proportion to my father's drinking.

Breakfast now included a quart of ice cream. Candy bar consumption nearly doubled, and I ate more sugar in a week than most people do in a year.

My brain function became even more severely compromised, and by the end of the summer I was regularly hearing voices.

"Barbara Altman, we're calling you. You're being watched."

Was sugar to blame? I still don't know. But according to my doctor, I'd become a Petri dish of yeast, mold, and fungus, and probably had a wildly erratic range of blood-sugar levels.

I was descending to a new level of depression, anxiety, and psychosis. The voices became more persistent and my hope for recovery plummeted.

Held captive in my own private jail, parole wouldn't come for many years.

CHAPTER TWELVE

In Jail: 1986, Age 42

My next assignment at the hospital was a visit to the minimum security area, followed by a three-day stint in maximum security. Each day we abandoned our identities and stepped through the gate from normalcy into a different reality of concrete and bars.

"Click" went the door as it closed on any semblance of sanity. During those sessions, I felt oddly secure, thanks to the alert guards and clean concrete-block cells.

Although she was probably only in her mid-twenties, the physically nondescript activities director, who took us to the main room, already had a rigid superior attitude and a highly developed talent for sarcasm and put-downs.

"See the prisoner at the card table?" She jabbed her stubby finger toward an innocent-looking man in his early forties, sitting comfortably with three other older men playing cards.

"You mean the choirboy-looking guy who's dealing now?" I ventured, focusing on the tall, good-looking man, who, even in his prison uniform, had the air of a competent businessman.

"That's him."

"What about him?"

"He murdered his wife and got a life sentence." She sneered, and I shivered. She had succeeded in scaring me half to death.

"I don't think I've ever met a murderer before!" I anxiously searched for the nearest exit. I wanted out of there quickly.

"Larned employs about a gazillion guards. You're probably safer here than you are anywhere else." She spoke the truth, and I began to feel secure there.

I spent the next three days in maximum security with the most serious offenders. The entire facility was gray and institutional inside and out. There were no frills, no plants, no brightly colored anything.

Several inmates worked on an art project, painting landscapes in watercolor. In contrast to the drab prison décor, the pictures danced with bright colors. Checking for the presence of guards, I nervously approached one of the artists and started up a conversation with a short, slim, bespectacled man, who looked pleased with his work.

"I like your painting. It's creative and unusual."

"Thank you. Every time I've been in prison, art class is my favorite activity," he said, concentrating on his brush stroke. *Every time?* I wondered if he enjoyed his re-imprisonments.

"Do you have an opportunity to market your work to the outside world?"

"No, we don't have that privilege," he shrugged. "However, when I'm released, I'll keep painting and try to sell my pictures." He continued to concentrate on his beginner-level painting.

I silently asked myself why he had repeated visits to prison. "Well, I really enjoy your work. Good luck to you."

On another visit, both Coreen and I had the opportunity to observe a music activity session, wherein the patients could choose among a dozen or more different records, all of which were traditional Sinatra-style vocals or sound tracks from musicals. The guard had to stay with us.

I introduced myself to a slightly overweight black man of average height with a look of naïve innocence on his face. He seemed out of touch with reality.

"I'm James. When I get out of here, I plan on becoming a scientist," he said gently.

I thought, *so far so good*, even if it did sound delusional.

"You have high goals for yourself." He seemed to want to make a large leap from prisoner to scientist.

"I do. I want to be a musician. I have connections in high places." His face brightened at the thought.

The hair stood up on the back of my neck, and I listened carefully to his words.

"I'm a personal friend of Ronald Reagan. He'll help me become an electrical engineer. I can make good money that way." He was becoming more and more excited. Eyes bulging, he talked on and on.

Something was terribly wrong. He had gone from science, to music, to electrical engineering, and from jail to the White House in seconds. He was a typical schizophrenic with fragmented language and delusions of grandeur.

All six men were sex offenders. That's why a guard had to be present. Had I known that, wild horses couldn't have dragged me into that room. Not a single one of them had the appearance of anything other than the average guy next door, showing no visual warning signs for those who came in contact with them. It brought to the surface powerful fears of being approached in a sudden, threatening manner. I stared at the ceiling and totally blanked out.

My mind went back twenty-seven years to the home I grew up in.

CHAPTER THIRTEEN

"The Three Faces of Eve:" 1958, Age 15

My mother and I, then fifteen, were watching, "The Three Faces of Eve," a movie about a woman who suffers from multiple personality disorder (see Section Two, Chapter One). They showed a flashback of three-year-old Eve being forced to kiss her dead grandmother. As a result, she suffered from post-traumatic stress disorder for most of her adult life. The movie was fiction based on a factual account said to have taken years of psychotherapy for her to become integrated into one functioning personality.

"You see," my mother said with empathy and sadness, "that child was traumatized. They should've never forced her to do that."

As had frequently happened, I remained silent, in a feeling state. An icy chill sent shock waves through my body. Why do I startle so easily when someone sneaks up on me? Why do I hear voices?

Shortly after this incident, I was in our kitchen with my father, talking about a former classmate who had just been arrested on eight counts of child molestation, accused of abusing several very young children.

I was numb at the thought of a grade school friend becoming such a monster.

"I can't believe he did such a horrible thing. It must be paralyzing to have sexual thoughts about young children."

"It is, Barbara, it is." Those five words seared my soul forever. My father always bellowed when he spoke, but this time he whispered like a haunted spirit.

I couldn't see him and didn't want to. I'd be happy if I never saw him again. I sat with my back to him wishing I'd never heard those words coming from my father's mouth – wishing I were dead.

What exactly had happened to me? I was fifteen years old and I couldn't pinpoint any specific memory, but I knew something traumatic had occurred to me as a very young child. In the deepest part of my being, I felt it.

So did something happen? Without having the memories, I can't prove it.

This I do know: We were having this discussion, one that no father and daughter should ever have.

We never again spoke to each other in any meaningful way.

I waited until he walked out the door and then I left.

CHAPTER FOURTEEN

Grandmothers, Mother, and Daughter: 1955 – 1958, Ages 12 – 15

The whole family (minus my father who was at work) had gathered at my dad's parents' home to celebrate his sister Annie's forty-fifth birthday.

My Altman grandparents lived in Baden, a St. Louis suburb of German immigrants, in a tiny stucco house filled with the comforting aromas of her cooking. All of her love and expertise went into the birthday cake and pot roast dinner. I never could decide who was the better cook, my maternal grandmother Tritz or paternal grandmother Altman.

My grandmother Tritz lived next door to us. I grew to two hundred pounds on her sugar doughnuts. I might have grown to three hundred pounds had Grandma Altman lived on the other side, baking her heavenly cinnamon apple strudel.

Sometime after Grandma had served her German chocolate cake, she began talking about my father.

Out of the blue, she said, "He came home drunk one day. I looked at him and yelled, 'Don't you ever do that again!' And he never did."

Short, round, and thoroughly German, she was shaking her finger and smiling with the recollection of her victory over his addiction.

I was about to explode. Damn! He's still drinking. He's wrecking the family! I'm constantly afraid of him.

I cried silent tears and stuffed a million tons of rage down my throat. I wanted to tell everybody about my father's passion for the bottle, but my mother gave me a powerful glare to say nothing. I was along in my pain and my need to blurt out the truth.

We all covered up for him, which added to his problems.

Grandmothers, mother, daughter – three generations of lost feminine power.

The same codependent drama played out with other women in the family. A few years later, my mother, Grandma Tritz, and I were in our kitchen waiting for my father, who was supposed to pick my grandmother up.

"Where's Ed? Why isn't he here?" She looked angry, sad, and hurt. "I'm already fifteen minutes late for my doctor's appointment! He's supposed to be here picking me up." Dressed in her tidy gingham housedress, my grandma, Eugenia Tritz, sat and sobbed.

"He's probably out drinking as usual!" My young voice shook with rage.

"Be quiet, Barbara!" my mother scolded, shooting enough death rays at me to nuke the universe.

Eugenia Rose Tritz had seen her own father dragged inside their home after an Iowa blizzard. He had gotten drunk, fell into the snow, and froze to death after a visit to the tavern. She saw his lifeless, frozen body. This dear woman lived to be ninety-two years old, never losing the sadness and pain when telling this story. I loved her with all my heart and I wanted to heal her emotional wounds.

Grandmothers, mother, daughter – three generations of women frozen by terror.

CHAPTER FIFTEEN

Teachers and Counselors at Larned: 1986, Age 42

After prison duty was over, I was assigned to the youth unit which housed six hundred or so teens and children of both sexes. There I observed a reading class of six teenaged boys in a small room where sports and car magazines lay on tables. In this activity, each boy was to select and read an article, and at the end of the session, had to answer a few questions designed to test their attention and comprehension.

They all fit the behavioral stereotype of youth at risk. I saw particular evidence of rebellion – the swagger, ever-present slouch, and belligerence, on the part of one young man.

That gangly young Kansas cowboy challenged the teacher. "Aw, dude, why the hell do I have to read this crap?"

"So they'll feed you dinner." Bob was burned out and counting the days to retirement. He, like his jeans and T-shirt, looked beaten and thoroughly worn out.

"Where do you get off telling me what to do?" the young cowboy sneered.

"You have to read it. So it would be a good idea to get on with it."

Instead of sitting down, the Kansas teen leaned against the wall and read the magazine, continuing to complain for the entire hour. But he got no further reaction from Bob, whom he knew couldn't care less if he read, as long as he shut up.

In contrast, the math class progressed smoothly. From her authoritative presence to her firm voice, Marie demanded their respect and attention.

I had a chance to talk to her briefly after the class.

"Your students seemed to enjoy the session." I wanted to learn how Marie was able to combine control of the class with compassion for each individual.

"I love my job. I'm due to retire in two weeks and I'll miss teaching." She looked away for a minute, and a look of sadness and loss crossed her face. "After that, I'd like to volunteer here a few hours a week."

After math and reading came a class of fifteen thirteen-year-old boys, all of whom had been sent there by the juvenile courts for behavioral counseling. Jason, their upbeat, vibrant counselor, knew each boy's family history by heart and talked about the unhealthy behaviors that had landed them in his classroom.

"This hospital is the last stop for those of you who've been busted," he told them. "If you break the law again, jail will be your next stop. And you really don't want that. Our Kansas courts are tough." As he stated the harsh facts, there was more than a trace of kindness in his voice.

He then passed out informational sheets about jobs and careers along with hourly salaries so they could all see what choices and venues they could choose from. Most of the jobs involved respectable, unskilled labor. Then he encouraged the boys to talk about their dreams and goals for the future, looking each one in the eye when they spoke and offering genuine smiles of encouragement as the students warmed to the topic. He gave them hope and vision, never allowing time for self-pity. The past is past. Now they're all about the future.

The positive energy in the room swelled, and I learned, too.

Teachers and counselors, they play a crucial role in a young person's life.

CHAPTER SIXTEEN

The Lunchroom: 1958, Age 15

My high school principal, Mother Gerard (a.k.a. Mother God), approached me as I stood in front of the tidy bulletin board, my eyes unfocused, stalling to avoid entering the lunchroom. "Barbara, why do you get stuck here every day instead of going in with the other girls?"

My gaze slid to the floor and my shoulders slumped. "No one ever wants to sit with me." My eyes welled up.

For the last year and a half, I had roamed the cafeteria, tray in hand, searching for a place to sit. My shyness and quiet manner made people uncomfortable, and I was often the butt of cruel jokes, like, "Here comes the space cadet." Day after day, I'd finally sit down and eat alone. I had almost convinced myself that I was better off being a free agent, sitting wherever I wanted, not tied to any particular group. Self-deception became my game. In those eighteen months, I hadn't made a single friend.

However, the day after Mother Gerard's comments, Rosalie Reddington, one of my classmates, came up to me outside the cafeteria. "Barbara, will you eat lunch with me?" A freckle-faced, red-headed, string bean of a girl, Rosalie was smart as a whip and a champion debater.

"Sure!" came my shocked response. We settled in at one of the tables, hardly talking. I was always silent, and she was probably a little ill at ease.

Despite her gesture of friendship, I still felt like a misfit. How painfully frustrating!

The next day, Eleanor asked me if I would join her and some friends for lunch. "What's going on?" I wondered, happy that at last my popularity ship was coming in.

And so it was that Eleanor, Sheila, Virginia, Ginny, and I ate together every day until we graduated. I would sit with them and let them hold up the conversation while I struggled not to let anyone see my brain fog and inner turmoil. What a blessing they were. Little did they know I was a candidate for a mental hospital.

It became routine. I would share that time with my four friends, only to then leave the cafeteria and walk down the very long hallway to the next class, jarred by wretched phantom voices coming from nowhere. They didn't bother me every day, but I never knew when they'd sound off.

As frightening as they were, the complete inability to concentrate felt more debilitating. The voices were sporadic, but the brain fog was constant and severe.

Trying to ignore it, I forced myself to focus on each and every word uttered by my teachers, one syllable at a time. But it's hard to learn that way, because you never get the big picture – just bits and pieces. I'm amazed I graduated and won a college scholarship to boot.

Every day, as soon as my last class ended, I would break down in exhausted sobs right there at my desk. Then after five or ten minutes of release, I'd pull myself together and go outside to wait for my dad to pick me up. Nobody ever stopped to ask me what was wrong. I think they were embarrassed.

Feeling heartbroken and desolate, I kept hoping for improvement.

I had to wait another forty years.

CHAPTER SEVENTEEN

Leaving Larned: 1986, Age 42

My remaining supervisor reviews at the hospital did not go well. Like a litany, week after week, Lanette would say, "You've got to let your hair down, greet people, look at us, and smile." I thought she was asking the impossible. How could I reinvent myself in just the first three weeks? I became even more withdrawn.

Anxious about succeeding or washing out of the internship, I foolishly showed up at activities employee Mary Williams's little white frame house one evening unannounced. Because she had always appeared kind, sociable, and very approachable, she seemed a safe outlet for my pent-up fear and frustration. What a terrible decision that was!

After at least an hour and a half of pouring my heart and tears out at her kitchen table, she abruptly stood up and said she needed to fix dinner. All I had picked up on was a slightly distressed look on her face. But I really had shot myself in the foot.

Mary was thoroughly distraught over my inappropriate visit, and the next morning she called Lanette to report my strange behavior. That, in addition to my overall inability to relate to staff and residents, provided the fuel needed to fire me.

As though this wasn't enough to get me the pink slip, I pulled one more trick. When my supervisor assigned a new patient to me, I was supposed to go to one of the brick residence buildings, pull his chart from the nurse's station, and work up a report summarizing his status and activity level. Thinking he might feel intimidated by having me look at his information, I marched up to the charge nurse and requested his records. She asked me who I was.

Now, I should have introduced myself as an intern from the activities department. Instead, thinking I was being assertive, I said, "You'll see."

News of that exchange traveled all over the facility like greased lightening. Lanette made the decision to let me go before I even got back to the activities building.

Assertive? That was plain rude. It came from years of poor socialization skills. I don't blame them for firing me. Ultimately, it became a real opportunity for change.

From the activities building just outside her office, I phoned Joan Shaw my music therapy mentor at Maryville University. Joan lives and breathes to encourage other people, and had guided me well during my two-year music therapy practicum at the Jewish Center for the Aged.

"Barbara, you can never be certain which internships will work out and which won't." Then her gentle voice became matter-of-fact. "Do you want a job?"

That practical question shifted me from despair to hope.

"Yes! Where?" I nearly jumped through the phone!

"There's one available at Bethesda-Dilworth Nursing Home as an activities aide for music therapy. She was sorting through papers on her desk to locate the right one.

What a gift that was! I'll always be grateful to Joan for making my transition from Larned back to St. Louis so much easier.

I reloaded my life into my steel gray Toyota Corolla, reversed directions, and headed home.

My six weeks at Larned had been both a wake-up call and a blessing. With Joan's help, I had a positive new direction.

CHAPTER EIGHTEEN

The Fontbonne Years: 1961 – 1965, Ages 17 – 21

My connection with Fontbonne College played a pivotal role in my life, beginning in my grade school years. When I was in fourth grade, my gloriously free-spirited, private music teacher, Betty Tyler, entered me into Fontbonne's annual music festival, as she did again in fifth and sixth grades. I dreamed of performing in the winners' concert and spent countless hours practicing to achieve that goal. (First place eluded me, but participating filled me with joy and self-pride.)

In this manner, the college served as a healing force and as a diversion from the challenges of my family. Not only did I receive the benefit of the "Mozart Effect," I also had a vital outlet. (The "Mozart Effect" is the positive effect of classical music on concentration.)

Whenever I'd become upset about my father's drinking and other troubling behaviors, I'd bring beauty into my life and to the world by going to my piano.

During my senior year in high school, I auditioned and applied for a music scholarship to Fontbonne College. My skilled presentation of a piece by Mendelssohn and one of the Beethoven Sonatas earned me first place, and in 1961, I began studying for my Bachelor of Music degree.

Music gave me solace, goals, and the tools necessary to build a life. I was gifted with a college degree, a career, and a place in the community. Fontbonne provided me a perfect milieu. All of us shared the same purpose. We were bonded by our interests and aspirations. I was taking classes I loved and was doing fine academically. Music majors tend to be outside-the-box creative people who understand a person's individuality.

My instructors treated me like everyone else. No one uttered the word, "schizophrenic," threatened me with institutionalization, or analyzed my behaviors to death. No longer living with the hateful label, my focus now shifted to my studies. I was simply Barbara.

I'd recovered from the worst part of the psychosis by my senior year. Of course, the most challenging aspect of my mental health continued to be brain fog.

The music and drama departments worked hand in hand each fall to produce their annual musical. I had a ball playing the piano in "Meet Me in St. Louis" and "Little Mary Sunshine" and was part of the chorus in "The Music Man". We had such fun during rehearsals and always had a cast party after productions. All this brought a welcome sweetness to my life.

The camaraderie with my friends and faculty members made those years so much more enjoyable. The laughter, hard work, and love for music may have precipitated the first stage of healing for me, for it was during my freshman year that I had my final hallucination (see Chapter Nineteen).

During my time at Fontbonne, I studied with Sister John Joseph Bezdek, head of the music department, whose sparkly good nature could turn to strict direction in a nanosecond. My first two years with her were challenging. I'd descended from being "Queen of the Hill" at the St. Louis Institute of Music to being an average, lowly freshman. Because I'd mastered the scales, arpeggios, and other exercises long since, I stubbornly refused to practice. In fact, I didn't do much of the assigned piano work, period. During my sophomore year, Sister Bezdek said unless I got to work, I wouldn't be able to attend the summer classes. That did it! I couldn't imagine that letter going home to my parents.

Besides, I was afraid of being kicked out and suffering the loss of my career dreams.

Once I began to buckle down to my piano studies, my love affair with that joy returned, and I played up a storm for three to four hours every day.

During my senior year, Sister Bezdek taught four of my classes and was tough in all of them. One day I approached her, saying, "Sister, I didn't do my counterpoint homework because I worked so hard at the piano." My stomach churned as I spoke. (Counterpoint refers to music written in the 18th century in the style of Bach. Our main project in that class was to write a vocal cantata in counterpoint.) Predictably, she replied, "I teach all four classes, not just one. You have to do the work in all of them"

I don't know why I thought she would change colors.

Throughout my college years, I never experienced any mollycoddling. If they suspected any mental illness, I wasn't aware of it. Their belief in my normalcy supported my healing.

Sister Bezdek set high expectations for all of us. When we did well, she never hesitated to compliment. I reached her goals on the piano, but not in her classroom, which frustrated her. But I did well enough to pass in spite of the rest of my problematic life.

She cut me no slack and pushed me upward toward higher and higher aspirations. Because of Sister Bezdek, I had goals to achieve. I had to stretch for the skies.

CHAPTER NINETEEN

Two Trips to Hell: 1961, Age 18

All of the music majors at my college had to participate in at least three choral concerts a year, comprised of classical vocal pieces and a few contemporary, 20th century classes. Although I loved singing, I hated those concerts because I would have one anxiety attack after another. We'd all file on stage with the top row first out of five. Being one of the tallest, I wound up right next to heaven. I dreaded standing there in my heavy black robe for an hour or more. With dry throat and stomach churning, I'd sweat and shake throughout the whole ordeal. But since our class grade depended on participation, I couldn't cop out.

One by one, I'd count off the pieces we sang. There would be fourteen songs, and then thirteen, twelve, until at last we were done. I fidgeted and squirmed during the entire performance. At the end, the midnight blue curtain would go down, we'd file off stage, and those on either side of me would support me by the elbows and walk me off. Even our director was concerned about my unsteady appearance.

For me, those concerts always culminated in tears.

At the end of each performance, all fifty women were fried from the hot lights, and one college freshman, me, was relieved to have survived that particular hell.

Our regular schedule of weekly choir rehearsals continued the following week with Sister still complaining about our section being flat. At every rehearsal, she said, "Altos, we need to sing that part over again. You're pulling all of us off key." Her usually twinkling eyes bored into mine.

I got a C in choir. I needed to maintain a B average in my music studies in order to keep my scholarship. So I tried to improve. Sister still glared in my direction. I made a strategic decision to either put up or shut up. I decided on the latter. For the next six months, I didn't sing one word. I became as non-singing as a female canary. Sister stopped nagging the altos, my grade went up to an A, and she even praised the improvement in my voice.

I had jumped two letter grades just by putting imaginary duct tape over my mouth.

By the end of my freshman year, my compassionate, overweight speech teacher, Carmelita Schmelig, could no longer overlook my constantly unkempt appearance and asked me if I would go with her to have my hair salvaged. Beauty parlor day arrived and she took me to an upscale salon located a few miles from the college.

"How do you want your hair done, Barbara?" inquired my gorgeous, blonde hair stylist.

"Make me look my best." Under my teacher's watchful eye, she proceeded to turn a sloppy teenager into a beauty queen.

Nearby, three other customers were having a gossip field day.

"Sally just had her baby . . . Did you hear about Susan? . . . Thelma and her husband . . ."

Consumed with my own concerns, I was only half listening. Watching the stylist sculpt my hair, I first felt like royalty and then became obsessed with my horrifying image.

I looked at myself in the mirror and beheld a heart-stopping, hideous hallucination. My face was distorted, with my eyes at the bottom and my mouth at the top. My ears sat at strange angles. I had no nose and my features were twisted to the left.

There were no words to describe the terror.

Miss Schmelig saw my anguish. "Barbara, are you all right?"

"I need to rest for a moment." I cupped my head in my hands, closed my eyes, and begged the vision to disappear. I couldn't tell her I'd just

hallucinated. That would be the end of my college career, my music studies, and the life I had planned for myself.

Then came the silent scream again!

Resolving not to utter one word about this, I hid in the closets of fear and shame. I looked gorgeous on the outside with beautifully coiffed hair, while my inner spirit collapsed.

"I have a little bit of stomach upset."

Clutching the counter, I'm imploding with rage and despair.

CHAPTER TWENTY

The St. Louis Institute of Music:
1969 – 1985, Ages 26 – 42

Following graduation, I worked for a year in Fontbonne's Preparatory Music Department teaching piano. Then I was hired at Washington University's Gaylord Music Library as a record librarian.

Beautiful tall buildings grace Washington University's ten-acre campus. The music library sits in a small enclave just opposite the medical school.

Located about ten miles <u>south</u> of Webster Groves, it was not within north *walking distance. Since I still didn't have a car, my father drove me to and from work. It didn't take long for my co-workers to learn about his drinking. To my shame and embarrassment, that news immediately spread around.*

The continuing pressures at home also affected my job performance. Unaware of the power of negative thoughts, I continued to bring my inner turmoil into the workplace.

After one year of uncontrollable and inappropriate crying spells and total disorganization, my boss called me into her office and fired me.

Groveling in shame, I felt like a complete and permanent failure, a nobody.

God had other ideas.

I was about to be rescued.

One sunny morning, synchronicity led me to Viola Grave's bookstore. I could have wandered into any one of the forty shops on Meramec Avenue in Clayton, but I chose the one with a job waiting for me.

Viola's shop was quaint, old, and emitted the aroma of musty, treasured books, all of which seemed wrapped in an aura of intrigue, mystery, and wisdom.

Tiny Viola, grey bun pulled tightly into a knot, greeted me warmly. "Good morning, Barbara. How can I help you today?"

"Do you have the Yellow Pages? I'm looking for employment agencies."

Wilma Kopecky, whom I'd known since my teen years, was sitting at her desk, typing up invoices. With her sharp mind, perfectly groomed hair, and stunning outfit, she personified my ideal woman.

"Didn't you go to the Institute of Music and study with Mrs. Mills?"

"Yeah. I studied with her in high school."

"Five teachers didn't sign contracts this year and Shirley Bartzen is desperately looking for replacements."

Dark eyes flashing, she stopped typing and looked me in the eye. "Thanks, Wilma!"

In my excitement, I dropped the ten-pound phone book splat on the floor, causing Wilma and Viola to look up in amazement.

Good-bye, Yellow Pages. It took one-half of one hot second to sprint into the alley and up the steps of the music school and into the next eighteen years of my life.

After one frantic knock, I burst into Shirley Bartzen's office, gulped air, and stammered, "I heard you're looking for piano teachers!"

Sitting at her desk, looking every bit the fashion model, she handed me an application, which I filled out in about two minutes.

My hire was confirmed within twenty-four hours and I was raring to go.

Shirley filled my roster with over fifty students.

I was no longer hallucinating, but still dealing with a high level of emotional sensitivity and brain fog. Although any hint of criticism still weighed on me like a ton of bricks, I had the perfect job.

Low self-esteem continued to plague me. My lack of good teaching skills resulted in frequent poor performances at student recitals. Many of my students didn't share my interest in the piano, and I lacked the nurturing skills to ignite their love of music. I tried to find the best teaching pieces and classics, but failed to teach them the basics. At the beginning of each school year, there were frequent requests from my students for a change of teachers. This pained me. Whenever my boss, Shirley, counseled me on these matters, I'd make corrections and things would go more smoothly. She called me into her office on a number of occasions to offer helpful advice and encouragement. To this day, I appreciate her kindness.

Though I was aware of my lack of teaching skills, some areas of my life brought satisfaction. My instrument, the piano, became a healing source. I fell in and out of love, I was active in my church, and I even managed a trip to Europe.

One afternoon, I got a notice that the president of the Institute of Music, J. P. Blake, wanted to see me in his office. Gadzooks! What did I do to merit this? What black mark had come to his attention?

At that time, we had to sign a contract stating that we would only use music published by the Art Publication Society, which was a sister business to the Institute. I had told one of my students to purchase some music at a music store.

This alone could've gotten me a pink slip.

I wondered if he was unhappy about my students' performances or if he knew about a lesson I'd forgotten. I walked in, sat in a chair opposite his desk, and awaited my doom.

But none of the above applied. Instead, he asked if I was interested in going on the annual school-sponsored trip to Europe. Feeling relieved, I signed up for a $2,000 trip to six European countries: Switzerland, Portugal, France, Italy, Germany, and Austria. Thus began my traveling adventures.

I also needed to get away. What a relief! Perhaps traveling six thousand miles from home would bring a different quality to my life.

CHAPTER TWENTY-ONE

European Adventures: 1970, Age 27

Departure date was June 6, 1970. After procuring the necessary passport and bundling up enough clothes to last at least a year in Europe, I boarded a plane for New York.

I called home as soon as I arrived in New York. My father was drunk when he took the call, so incapacitated he could hardly talk. His drinking haunted me 900 miles away! Not even Europe could erase that reality.

In the days and weeks prior to my departure, he continued to scream at me routinely, usually over things that were of no consequence. The intensity of his voice brought fear, shame, and anger to my heart. He would yell out of his own frustration and rage.

That trip presented such a welcome break. I had three weeks of not being harassed and not having to hear or see an alcoholic parent. He was drunk and screaming the day of my departure and the day of my return. I wished I had an ally who would've helped me figure out a way to get out of there so I could build a life independent of his problems.

Now six thousand miles away from home I still carried a heavy load of fear, and the plane ride itself terrified me. In fact, when I boarded the 747 headed for Geneva, Switzerland, I knew what to expect.

People suffering with anxiety need to meet threatening situations in tiny increments. There was no way of desensitizing myself to my height phobia. Jumping out the window wasn't an option. I had to sit there and bear it.

It helped to close my eyes for a few seconds at a time. In that way, I gradually achieved enough calm to remain intact for the rest of the seven-hour trip.

Once in Switzerland, my group took a trolley ride up Mount Pilatus. Thirty-two of us ascended to the top. Thirty-one of us thoroughly enjoyed it. I nearly died. I just about tore the metal handhold in two with the strength of my grip.

Oh, how I wished I wouldn't feel such terror and dissociation whenever my body rose more than three feet off the ground. Why couldn't I be carefree like everyone else? What about me? When would it be my turn? Nevertheless, I managed to take gobs of pictures of Swiss chateaus from the trolley. Sometimes I amazed myself. Who else would have pushed past all that fear to take photos?

The trek up was worth it. Staying about one hundred feet back from the edge forestalled a panic attack. What beauty we saw: storybook, snow-capped mountains as far as the eye could see. It was worth every moment of the ride up.

I'll never forget it.

During our first week in Switzerland, an angel was watching over me. One evening, at my roommate's urging, I pulled my long black evening gown with the sassy, sexy slit out of the closet, got all dolled up, and walked to a dance at the hotel next door.

There I entered a classic dance scene complete with a dimly-lit ballroom, a bar, and the flicker of psychedelic lights coming from a lighted mirror ceiling. In spite of the enchanted setting, my prince charming failed to show, and I left four hours later.

Two men followed me as I walked out the door. One of them left while the other continued to follow. He grabbed me by the arm as we were walking between hotels and forced me to kiss him.

I planned on screaming if no one was in the hotel lobby. Sure enough, it was empty. I was getting ready to yell at the top of my lungs, when I looked toward the staircase and saw five men from my tour party coming down the steps.

My abuser bolted out the door to the street. I almost collapsed from sheer relief.

Feeling enormously grateful, I asked them what on earth they were doing roaming around the hotel at 1:30 in the morning.

"Anna Maria sent us out to look for you."

Anna Maria, our psychically-gifted tour friend, had had a nightmare vision of my life-threatening attack. She became hysterical and woke our tour guide, Dick Kaufmann, pleading and demanding that they search for me.

"You've got to go find Barbara. She's in serious trouble."

All six of us shared a heartfelt group hug.

Those five men probably saved my life that evening and that experience convinced me I had a guardian angel watching over me.

But the excitement wasn't over yet.

A few days later, we were scheduled to take a bus ride up Mount Bergt in Lucerne, driving right into an ice and snow storm. Although the weather forecast called for light snow in the mountains, we got at least ten inches. The farther up the mountain, the worse the weather was. My intuitive friend, Anna Maria, told us she wasn't going to be completing the trip. She'd had a premonition about some sort of accident.

The bus slid around icy curves as the weather continued to deteriorate. Finally, the driver and the tour guide told us to stay in our seats while chains were being put on all eight tires. Everyone protested. The last place we wanted to be was on that bus. We were 14,000 feet up and the driver was repeatedly jockeying the bus toward the edge of the mountain to get the chains adjusted. Of course, I was sitting next to the drop. Of course!

Rosaries were flying furiously, especially Anna Maria's. "Oh, my God!" someone yelled. "One more inch and we're going over the side."

"Shut up!" someone else shouted.

I was clearly suffering, saying my prayers as swiftly and earnestly as the others said their rosaries.

From behind me, Martha offered her motherly sarcasm. "Calm down, Barbara. You look white as a sheet. We're going to be okay. The driver probably has had a lot of experience with these situations."

Despite this assurance, I felt I was spinning out of control, but for once, I wasn't the only one.

"Don't look down, Barbara, and you won't be so scared." Martha wasn't very helpful.

I looked straight ahead. It didn't help. My acute anxiety disorder magnified the terror.

Somehow, thankfully, we made it through without plummeting over the edge.

After three weeks of travel, we had to return home. Despite my various frightening experiences, I didn't want to go back. Realistically, I had little choice. My freedom from the stresses of home life had ended and it was time to go back to the hellhole of home.

I arrived home pumped up from my trip, vowing to return to Europe. Actually, I just yearned to get out of that house and move as far away as possible.

"I want to take some foreign language classes so I can travel again." I was full of happy prospects for the future.

"Shut up, Barbara! You just got back!" my father screamed at me with his abusive tone of voice.

Welcome back, I thought to myself. My bliss was over. Say hello to the world of hopelessness. Alcoholics bring despair to their families. I now had been exposed to five men on the tour who treated me with respect. Absent were my father's routine tantrums.

All my life I had been living in "One Flew Over the Cuckoo's Nest," but now knew how functional people behave with each other.

CHAPTER TWENTY-TWO

Confrontation: 1973, Age 30

Forgiveness is a key component of every world religion.

The week-long Christian seminar at Melodyland Christian Church in Anaheim, California, convinced me to turn my problems over to God. Several hundred upbeat individuals and I learned to turn confrontation into the opportunity for forgiveness. I returned home super-charged with intention.

The very next day, my father erupted into a screaming fit. And my crime? I opened the refrigerator to get a glass of milk. I was thirty years old at the time.

Eyes bulging and face crimson, he again treated me like an imbecile.

"Oh, stay out of there. We're going over to Red Lobster in a few minutes. What the matter with you?"

My heart sank. "What's the matter with you?" was such a trigger for me.

"There's nothing wrong with me!" I declared through my tears.

Finally, I decided not to suffer in silence. I went to my room, read my Bible, prayed to calm myself, and figure out how to approach him.

With my new-found resolve and my heart in my throat, I asked my father to come into the living room where we could talk.

Finally, I broke my twenty years of silence. "Dad, I know that I haven't been the daughter that you've wanted me to be, and I apologize for that." Actually, I had no reason to apologize, but I had an insatiable urge to demean myself. "But I want to know why you yell at me so much. That really hurts. And I don't like your drinking. I want you to stay out of the taverns." Nearly choking on the tears and anguish, I put more than two decades of suffering into my words.

My father suddenly looked stunned and utterly defeated.

"Don't you know how much I love you?" Tears glistened in his eyes. "I go to the taverns to gamble and make money. I do it all for you so you won't have to worry about money."

"I don't care about the money. All I've ever wanted is the real you to come back home. When you choose the bars over us, I feel worthless and completely unlovable." I spoke with restraint while turmoil raged inside me.

"How can you talk about loving me?" I asked. "Love is demonstrated by where your heart is, and it seems like yours in at the tavern."

Tears ran down his face.

He was clueless about the effect drinking had on all of us! I really felt angry. How could he be so numb to our pain?

CHAPTER TWENTY-THREE

Bethesda-Dilworth: 1986, Age 42

I continued to teach at the St. Louis Institute of Music, which merged with the Community Music School to become St. Louis Conservatory and School for the Arts, known as CASA. For me, the same challenges remained.

Yes, I had a few stellar students, but my overall job performance left much to be desired. Well aware of my inadequacies, I worried about job security. Knowing that studying the classical composers had been such a healing force for me, I decided to pursue the study of music therapy. I limped through my teaching years, continuing to produce mediocre results, and, in 1982, made the transition to my new career choice at Maryville University.

There I embarked upon the two-and-a-half years of training needed to qualify for the internship experience at Larned State Hospital, which, of course, ended prematurely after six weeks.

As the saying goes, "All things work together for the good of those who love the Lord."

Put more graphically, even manure can make good fertilizer.

Being fired was about as appealing as pond scum. I was devastated. But God and I had something else on the back burner; a new venture was about to begin.

The long drive home from Larned gave me the opportunity to review my life. Not happy with what I saw, I set a firm intention to do a major overhaul on my personality. It no longer served me to keep my eyes on the floor when greeting someone. My experiences in Kansas inspired me to liven up my act a bit.

At Bethesda-Dilworth Nursing Home, I had time on my side since each new employee had a six-month trial period. I could accomplish my goals at a comfortable pace. Positive change was now a part of my thinking.

During my first job review at the home, my supervisor, Lynne Weigert, made comments about my looking "zoned out."

I felt so disappointed! Damn! Not enough change yet! I had to adjust or lose my job.

Lynne personified the ideal supervisor. Organized, supportive, and kind, she is also physically beautiful with black hair, brown eyes, and alabaster skin.

"Barbara, I've seen you in the hallway several times looking lost. When I first started working here, I made a map of the facility so I'd know exactly where I needed to be every minute of the day.

Did my supervisor at Larned communicate with my boss at the nursing home? They both had the same language with regard to my behavior. Curse that work "lost." How it made me cringe! I knew I had to take action if I didn't want to keep hearing it. I now had the incentive to begin correcting this situation. Fortunately, my boss continued to offer me useful suggestions.

"Barbara, we want you to ask more questions. You seem to be reluctant to participate. At staff meetings, you're too quiet and passive. We want you to be involved with the process and to contribute to our discussions."

Evidently, I bugged people at both Larned and Bethesda.

Sweet Lynne gave me another chance by putting me on probation, after which I'd be reviewed again.

It was time to get more proactive in my healing. I set up an appointment with counselor Ray Fezzi at St. Louis Family and

Children's Services. I chose that route because of my positive experience there six years earlier with Patricia Antle.

I bought a tally counter and used it to track each of my positive interactions with others.

Eye contact had always been a challenge. Looking at the ground served me well for forty-two years, but now I needed to move on. I had become shy, introverted, and lacked confidence. Casting my gaze downward protected me from feeling invaded and violated.

Once I bought my counter, I gave myself one click every time I said "hello" to someone, two clicks if I smiled, and three clicks if I looked up. Oh, and I got fifty clicks if I talked to a man. I hid my little gray clicker in my pocket so it would be less obvious.

Fingers flying deftly over the gadget, I set goals for myself. Forty clicks got me a new blouse, fifty was cause for getting a new dress, and one hundred merited a new coat. I managed to earn about enough clicks to purchase a fancy, white, silk blouse.

I used this technique freely at Bethesda, which was the perfect environment since I had a captive audience. Many of the residents had a limited use of vocabulary and were wheelchair bound. What an ideal training ground!

The mirror became a friend! Standing in front of it, I would smile, laugh, scrunch up my face, and frown. What fun I had, becoming a contortionist! That flat affect had to go!

After a few minutes in front of my mirror each morning, I felt ready to go to work.

Observing and connecting with my surroundings and the people I served continued to create healthy interactions.

"Good morning, Mrs. Smith. What a pretty, blue housecoat you have on!"

"My back hurts. The nurse just gave me some medicine and it hasn't kicked in yet." Ella Smith had a little sassy streak.

"Hang in there. The medicine will start working soon." I actually looked at her and smiled. How novel! My cheeks were beginning to crack with the strain of an expression.

Through such interactions, I would eventually earn my silk blouse.

With a spring in my step, I headed for the activities room where more clicking opportunities awaited.

Small successes were becoming easier, but I still had to concentrate on livening up my facial expressions.

Brief exchanges were no longer a hurdle; whereas, keeping the conversation going continued to be painful and frustrating.

It helped to observe healthy people. One doesn't have to be talkative to keep words and conversation going at a good clip. Nodding appropriately, smiling, looking interested, and, most importantly, using active listening skills contributed as much as the words did.

Positive results slowly began to creep in.

One novel incident in particular stands out in my mind.

The singles group at my church went out to lunch every Sunday after the service. I was talking with one of the men who seemed to hang onto my every word. I thought it must have been some sort of fluke. I kept talking, wondering if it was my imagination, when I saw the same look of animation on his face. Was I dreaming?

Relishing the chance to return the compliment, I piped up, "Larry, tell me about the cabinet-making trade. How do you find the time to deal with all of your customers?" His response genuinely interested me.

"I love my trade and I've become adept at handling more than one job at a time."

"I'm impressed. How long have you been doing that?"

"I started in the cabinet- and furniture-making business right after college, which was about twenty-five years ago."

This conversation went on for about forty-five minutes, which was a record for me and demonstrated that hope loomed on the horizon at long last. I was beginning to feel whole.

This new-found skill made its way into my job at Bethesda; communication became easier.

I saw quantitative results in my job review. At my next review, my supervisor removed probation. Thank you, Lynne Weigert. My hard work with therapist Ray Fezzi was really paying off.

CHAPTER TWENTY-FOUR

Music Therapy with the Elderly: 1998, Age 55

When I began working as a music therapist at a local nursing home in 1998, I had the responsibility of leading groups on the floors. We would do Mitch Miller-style sing-alongs, rhythm band, and talk about the music. Every class was built around a theme, such as flowers or something seasonal, and everyone relished concluding the sessions with a rousing John Phillip Sousa march. The residents practically danced out of their wheelchairs.

I opened with a welcoming song, usually "Hail, Hail the Gang's All Here," followed by greeting each resident by name and savoring their smiles of happy anticipation. Next came some mild exercises and deep breathing routines. Then I would lead the singing and rhythm band.

Energized by their new-found musical skills, they filled the room with joy.

Mary always played the cowbell to the tune of "I've Been Working on the Railroad." She'd clang out the beat to the accompaniment of the piano, bells, and rhythm sticks.

After each session, Mary telephoned her husband, Bill, to tell him, "The music lady was here today and I got to play the cowbell. She let me lead the choir when we sang."

Because of her bipolar disorder, she got out of bed only for mass, meals, and music. But for "music class," she even put on lipstick.

Mary died about two years ago. Her husband was in the rehab section recovering from a fall, and I had the opportunity to give him the beloved cowbell. It now holds a place of honor in their home on top of her piano.

It felt like I was doing what I was born to do in serving the elderly.

My time at the two senior facilities where I currently work is devoted to bi-weekly, one-on-one music therapy sessions. I have the privilege of visiting the dearest of the dear, the oldest of the old, and the neediest of the needy.

One special gift the elderly give us is the opportunity to learn and practice compassion, allowing their caretakers to work together as a team. At the nursing home, I see a place full of love and concern for those who have cared for others. Now it's their turn.

Down the hallway, I passed by the room of a former Lindbergh School District superintendent, Robert Allen, who had recently died, and I paused to softly sing a good-bye to him. After one last song, I walked out, remembering the music sessions we'd had over the past eighteen months and felt grateful for having known him.

Robert Allen is still lovingly honored in the Lindbergh School District and surrounding area.

In my new-found, more sociable mode, I exchanged normal pleasantries with co-workers as I continued my rounds, visiting a few more residents before completing my two-hour shift.

When I stopped by to see Alma, I saw pain and fear in her wrinkled face.

"Hi, Alma. How are you doing today?" giving her an opening to share.

"I'm scared," she said, speaking through her tears. "I don't know which end is up. I'm so frightened. I keep seeing bugs crawling on the walls and the ceiling. My father died in an insane asylum and I've always been afraid I'd go insane, too."

She went on to tell me that a new arthritis medication seemed to be causing frequent hallucinations, and she didn't know whether to focus on her pain or on mental clarity. Alma was ninety-eight.

"I understand your fear, Alma. Trust me, you have my sympathy." All too well did I understand.

Many years before, my mother and I went downtown to shop for school clothes on one of the few days she had available for the task. We got off the bus somewhere on Kingshighway and waited for the connecting bus to take us to our destination.

I looked up to the sky and watched in horror as every building around me grew and grew and grew to unimaginable heights. Feeling lightheaded and frightened, I spotted a dumpster nearby. The world had gotten too much for me to handle, and in desperation, I slumped to the ground, clutched it, and wept.

"What's wrong, Barbara?" I heard real alarm in my mother's voice.

"I don't feel well."

"We have to shop today. It's the only time I have to buy those clothes."

"I can't go on. I want to go home."

Feeling as though I could not endure life for one more second, I clung to that old dumpster with every ounce of fear in me. Why did I have to experience such terror? Would life never be any different? Would I live like this forever?

I couldn't move. It was all too hard. I wanted to give up. I was tired, so tired that death would have been a welcome release.

We got on the bus and headed back to Lizette Avenue. Again, I sucked it all up, only confessing to feeling sick. We arrived home and celebrated my grandmother's birthday as though nothing unusual had just happened.

CHAPTER TWENTY-FIVE

My Father's Final Years: 1972 – 1976, Ages 29 – 33

Years of drinking finally took a toll on my father's body and his health slowly declined. In 1972, at age seventy-three, he began to feel weak and run down. Although never one to go to a doctor, he finally admitted to being ill and made an appointment with Dr. Frank Manganaro. There he was diagnosed with myelofibrosis and cirrhosis of the liver, both the results of his excessive alcohol consumption.

He had a difficult time facing his mortality. He often wept, devastated by remorse and profound regret over the lost years. My father would sit in his favorite leather chair, cup his face in his hands, and mourn his life.

As he struggled to accept his fate, he continued to bargain. "Please, dear God, I promise to try to make up to my family for all the hurt I caused if you just let me live long enough to see my grandchildren grow up."

One afternoon he found a picture of me with several grade school classmates.

"Barbara, I missed out on so much of your life. If only I could take back those years. I didn't know about those friends of yours. I'm so sorry." And he sobbed.

"I didn't have close relationships, Dad. I felt lost. Most of the time I had to search for friends to share lunch with at school. I felt like an outcast." My pent-up rage spewed out.

If I'd been more confrontational, I might've said, "No, we weren't close at all. Any chance of a loving childhood bond is long gone. You didn't live up to your role as a father. I rarely invited friends over because I dreaded your embarrassing behavior."

Ignoring his impending death, I remained in denial up to the end. The fires of rage and sadness nearly consumed me.

During that dying time, his irascible temper knew no bounds. The screaming episodes grew in frightening intensity. The reality of his decline exacerbated the emotional chaos that had defined his life.

I felt defeated, depressed, and oppressed. A balanced father-daughter relationship seemed beyond us. I ricocheted between loving him and hating his actions.

His physical deterioration accelerated rapidly. After four years of intense suffering, he was admitted to Deaconess Hospital in October 1976. I still couldn't face facts, even though death was his constant companion.

Walking down the hallway one day, I saw an emaciated old man slouching in a wheelchair. Thinking no one that close to death should be alone, my heart ached for the elderly gentleman.

I came within six feet of him before recognizing my own father. With a start, I realized I had felt more compassion for the stranger than for him, and my heart softened for my dad. That speaks volumes.

He looked up at me. "Barbara, I'm so glad to see you." He seemed broken. When did he grow old? I could no longer deny the reality of his coming death.

Three days later, as my mother and I sat in the hospital cafeteria eating dinner, we heard a code blue for the sixth floor. "That's your dad," she said. We both jumped up and ran for the elevator.

I sat outside his room with my mother trying to take it all in.

In a flurry of activity several nurses and doctors fought to revive him. All at once they all stepped back from his bed. One of the doctors, I don't remember which one, came out and spoke to us.

"We did everything possible for him. He died about two minutes ago. Would you like to go see him?"

Nothing prepared me for what I experienced. We can glamorize death all we want. It just isn't pretty. His lifeless body was turning ashen and stiff. The utter stillness of death sent a chill into the air.

The coldness of this experience could be matched only by the dysfunction in our relationship. As he lay there so still and quiet, I prayed for peace in his next life. I can't say I've ever felt sorry for him, but I've felt sadness for the incomplete us.

My mom let me go in first. I touched his lifeless hand and sat at his bedside. In rapid-fire succession, scenes of the pain and abuse in his early life and the mixed pride, fear, and anger I felt in our relationship flashed through my mind. The guilt that swept through me at the release of his death colored the sadness of what now never could be.

CHAPTER TWENTY-SIX

My Mother's Final Years: 1992 – 1995: Age 49 – 52

My mother and I were polar opposites. She was the quintessential extrovert; I was introverted and introspective. She had a warm, effusive personality; I did not. She had the gift of gab; I'd be shocked if anyone happened to listen to anything I said. I drew energy from her essence.

I felt dwarfed by her presence and loved her. What would I do without her?

After her heart surgery in 1984, her doctor told her to exercise, which she did religiously, often taking long walks. Easter Sunday 1992 was a beautiful day. I was driving home from church, when I spotted my mother, ashen and pale, walking toward me. She looked frightened.

I helped her into the car and took her home.

She'd come down with diarrhea and suffered other flu-like symptoms until she got a prescription about a week later. But she continued to become more and more confused, and my family and I noticed frequent episodes of memory loss.

Because of the gradual deterioration, I set up a neurological evaluation with a local psychiatrist.

The diagnosis was grim – Alzheimer's. Both of our worlds fell apart and my mother's insidious march toward her death began. By now I'd had enough exposure to the ravages of this disorder to know the prognosis. Still, I wasn't prepared for what was to come.

Shortly after that, Mother started getting up in the middle of the night to leave the house! One morning, at about 2:30 a.m., I was awakened by her sister, Alma, who was trying to stop her from walking out the front door.

"I have to go out and take my walk. The doctor says if I don't exercise, my heart condition will get worse." She was sitting at the kitchen table fully dressed in her white walking shoes and blue pants suit.

"Mom, you can't go out the door in the middle of the night!"

"Yes, I can! I have to walk!" She was yelling at the top of her lungs.

Her voice was typical of an Alzheimer's patient who's in the middle of a catastrophic event, an occurrence characterized by an outburst of temper that's often precipitated by sensory overload. The more we tried to bring her back to reality, the more agitated she became. She had her own agenda.

I decided to take a different approach. I went to the telephone, picked it up, and set it back down again.

"Mom, I just talked to the doctor. He's advising you to eat something first."

I went to the refrigerator, pulled out some vanilla ice cream, and we all proceeded to have a 2:45 a.m. snack. This seemed to satisfy her. After all, it was the "doctor's orders." By the time she finished eating, she had forgotten all about the walk. It was a technique I'd learned from my years of work in nursing homes.

Her anxiety was more than matched by mine. In the beginning, she was aware of her frequent memory loss. She'd look at me with tears in her eyes and wonder why she couldn't remember things any more.

Those outbursts, periods of intense anger, and high anxiety became more frequent as her disease progressed. My mother expressed her feelings with temper tantrums and screaming fits whenever she couldn't get her point across.

Tensions ran high. Since I'd made the commitment to keep her out of a nursing home, I hired caretakers around the clock to deal with the situation. Overseeing her care was a demanding, stressful job. Once again, one-on-one counseling helped me through.

In my weekly sessions, my therapist listened to me pour out my feelings and frustrations. Her support and encouragement sustained me. She insisted I take regular breaks from my caretaking routines.

Following her advice, I visited Pere Marquette State Park on the last weekend of each month. Overlooking the confluence of the Mississippi and Illinois rivers, I relaxed, read, hiked and enjoyed the scenery.

Once again, my spiritual connection with God, together with my family and the resources available in the mental health community, became lifelines for me.

When my mother was first diagnosed, the family met at my nephew's home. Together, we devised a plan to help her during her final illness. My nephews installed handrails and put up motion detectors so I'd know when she'd awaken in the middle of the night. This was before I hired the full-time caretakers.

Our first caretakers came on board about three months later. I hired Joyce Hurst from Lutheran Senior Services and she recommended Lena Johnson and several of her friends, all of whom took care of my mother on a 24/7 basis.

Joyce spent up to one hundred hours a week in our home and Lena worked three morning shifts. They fed, clothed, and entertained my mother. She was kept occupied with simple mathematics books, movies, and television. Mom always loved arithmetic. Once a week, one of us drove her to Douglas Manor where she played bingo, socialized with other seniors, and ate lunch. My mother, always the extrovert, enjoyed the company.

My decision to keep my mother at home was firm. I couldn't bear the thought of dropping her off at a facility and looking back as I'd leave. She loved her house and I feared the change would kill her. Of course, in retrospect, I realize those concerns weren't realistic. She could always adjust to new situations.

I, on the other hand, wasn't willing to adapt. My mother's presence and energy had been a source of strength for me all of my life. I couldn't rip myself from her.

Watching her change from a quick-witted person to a slow-moving victim made me ache for her, and I hated her harsh, relentless transformation.

In spite of all that, her final years also included times of joy and peace. She learned to find fulfillment in the simple acts of life. She sang, played dominoes and slapjack, and adored talking, hugging, and above all, smiling.

My mother's illness was characterized by many of the same mental problems that I'd experienced as a teenager. She suffered from hallucinations and depression. Years before, I'd lost my vision for a future and my will to live. She was looking at death and her disease took her life.

During the last six months, she had traumatic flashbacks of her life with my father. I used to hold her and sing to her to quiet her down. She'd scream and cry out, "They shouldn't do that to me! They shouldn't do that!"

One evening, just before she fell asleep, I heard her whimpering, "I didn't want to go out with him. I didn't even want to see him. I was dating someone else and I didn't like him!" She was so inconsolable that it took nearly an hour to calm her down.

Through her painful situation, we experienced beautiful healing together. For thirty years, I'd been aware of my mother's very negative reaction to the news of her second pregnancy – with me. Apparently, her anger knew no limits. She'd been seeing a chiropractor who corrected her tilted uterus, but neglected to tell her to use protection. She got pregnant.

Knowing this made me feel like an unwanted intruder until my fifty-first birthday. I was driving her home from the hospital after one of her many visits. This time she'd been kept in restraints for three days and was screaming, "Don't tie me up!" from the moment we got into the car, over and over.

In an effort to distract her and keep us both safe on the road, I tentatively said, "Mom, today's my birthday."

"Happy birthday, Barbara."

"How did you feel fifty-one years ago today?"

I was nervous, knowing Alzheimer's patients speak candidly and don't filter their responses.

"That was the most beautiful baby. I fell in love with her right away." That statement melted away years of uncertainty in my heart.

I'd always been angry that she stayed with my father in spite of the pain he caused his family. She also spoke of this during her illness.

One afternoon I found her outside, sitting in her favorite green lawn chair, crying her eyes out. "I should've left him. I didn't leave him and God is punishing me by making me sick," she moaned.

"Do you think God is mad at you?" I felt a tender mix of annoyance and compassion.

Then I spoke up. "Actually, to be honest, Mom, I've always been angry with you because you chose to stay."

She looked at me with tears in her eyes and began to smile. "Will you forgive me?"

How could I not forgive her?

"You know I do, Mom," and I put my arms around her as I said those words.

My mother and I had two healing rituals. I used to hug her several times a day, saying, "I love you as high as the sky and back."

"I love to hear you say that, Barbara," she beamed. I believe the deepening affection we felt for each other helped to extend her life.

Singing the old favorite, "Show Me the Way to Go Home," became our routine good-night song. It had to be sung or she wouldn't go to sleep. The tide had turned. Just as she used to soothe me with lullabies, I now comforted her with music.

On the evening of February 16, 1995, we shared our nightly song just before she went to sleep. The caretakers had Thursdays off so it was just Mom and me.

She awoke at 1:15 a.m. coughing up heavy phlegm.

"Why can't I sleep?"

I went into the bathroom to get some Kleenex.

"Thank you, honey. You're so sweet."

When I returned, she was no longer responding. She'd had a massive heart attack. About ten minutes later, four paramedics arrived and struggled to bring her back to life. She was taken to St. Mary's Hospital where she died at 3:45 p.m. on February 17, 1995.

The nurses came into the waiting room and asked me if I wanted to go in and see her. I asked for privacy, held her dear hand, and sang to her one last time.

After two and a half years of suffering from Alzheimer's, she had at last gone home.

I loved my mother. We had difficult times, but the nature of our relationship was one of a mutual bond, a strained, but loving link. Her last years held both joy and stress. Fortunately, I was supported by my family, my mother's caretakers, Lena and Joyce, my faith, and my therapist. They were all part of my support group and they enabled me to maintain my equilibrium while I entered into the task of her care.

CHAPTER TWENTY-SEVEN

Trying to Heal My Body:
1987 – 1989, Ages 43 – 45

It was time to explore whole-body healing and I decided to look into alternative methods. Unfortunately, my "doctor" nearly killed me.

Brain fog, from which I still suffered, is complex to explain. One's thought processes are deadened, thwarted, and compromised. Although there's a strong body-mind connection, I spent years living on the edge, with one foot in the normal world and the other in the reality of a compromised mind.

What a lonely experience! Millions have colds, heart attacks, or depression. But I despaired of finding anyone who had experience treating brain abnormalities, and believing sincerely that no doctor would be able to help me, I bore its horror alone for more than thirty-three years.

This would be my "cross," my path to redemptive suffering, or so I thought.

I lived in a crappy world!

While the behavioral techniques I'd learned became essential to my recovery, I needed to get my body to cooperate. One can't maintain a lively affect if the brain is functioning at half mast.

So I became motivated to seek answers to my physical problems. From 1987 to 1989, between the ages of forty-three and forty-five, and on the recommendation of a friend, I had weekly visits to a naturopathic "doctor."

Her advice proved to be dangerous and almost deadly. Ms. Jones was a blot on the reputation of all honorable naturopaths.

Too bad I ignored my first impression. Seventy-five miles from my home, in very rural Missouri, she and her spouse and their seven children lived in little more than a shanty with goats grazing in their front yard.

Feeling so sick and desperate, I was grasping at straws and chose to ignore my gut reaction.

I was advised to eat a vegan diet of only raw foods, with no instructions about effective protein building. I was to eat one fruit meal per day.

However, this fed indirectly into my sugar addiction as mentioned in Chapter Eleven.

I turned to fruit to balance out my feelings, substituting apples and bananas for candy bars.

Lunch might consist of five apples, two bananas, and six dates. Needless to say, my sugar levels bounced off the wall.

Already slender at one hundred and thirty pounds on a five-foot-eight frame, I dropped to ninety-five pounds and entered into full-fledged anorexia. But my naturopath told me to remain on the diet or I'd die.

My friends said I looked like an Auschwitz survivor. My mother was terrified. So was I.

Ms. Jones made one serious mistake, almost costing me my life.

I have a thyroid that is seriously inactive. During one of my weekly visits, I discussed my situation with her.

"Dr. Jones, I'm concerned about taking such a large dose of these thyroid meds (which had been prescribed by a different health-care provider). I read about the negative effects of prolonged thyroid replacement on heart function."

She said, "Can it. If you continue with your diet and the recommended herbs, your thyroid will balance out."

Unfortunately, I took her advice. About three weeks later, I was on a dinner date at C.J. Muggs in Webster Groves. While there, I began to feel weak, woozy, and disoriented.

We left the restaurant and bowled a couple of games at a local alley. On the way out the door, I passed out and bashed my head against the wall.

Dazed, confused, and bloody, I didn't regain consciousness until the ambulance was on its way. I was afraid I was dying. At St. Anthony's emergency room, I got eleven stitches just above my left temple.

They released me into my mother's care with strict instructions that I wasn't to be left alone for at least twenty-four hours. My sweet mother sat vigil at my bedside all night so I wouldn't drop off to sleep unattended.

My naturopath called herself a "healer." She has since been sued for fraud by the same friend who recommended her.

Frightened about weight loss, I felt trapped as I remembered her prediction of death. Of course, continuing down the same road was killing me anyway. Which way should I turn?

What anguish gripped my soul! Damned if I did and damned if I didn't! Darkness loomed in my thoughts. I wept non-stop.

Trying to manage my situation alone no longer worked. Worried about my health, brain fatigue, and an assortment of other concerns, there was no corner of life that felt comfortable. No joy, satisfaction, or direction entered my thinking. The incident at the bowling alley became a call to pursue counseling.

It took intensive mental health intervention to bring me to a point of change.

SECTION 1
Part Two

Creating the Will to Live:
My Journey Toward Healing

And Caroline said,
"Barbara, how much do you want to live?"
I remained silent.
"I'll understand that to mean you don't want to survive."
I set the intention to fan the flames of life.

CHAPTER TWENTY-EIGHT

Therapy – Creating the Will to Live: 1989, Age 46

My new life began the day I walked in psychologist Caroline Penberthy's office. As she opened the door, my first thought was, *at last, someone taller than me*. At the recommendation of a friend, I had called Caroline to introduce myself and make an appointment.

"I have a concern because I have a problem with overeating and a kaleidoscope of other issues." That conversation occurred the day after I was released from the hospital with eleven stitches on my head. I weighed ninety-five pounds.

Her initial greeting was, "We have to get some weight on you!"

I assumed I would see her for about six months, deal with my "overeating" problem, and then move on with my life. Was I in for a shock!

Caroline had short gray hair, large expressive blue eyes, and an obviously gentle spirit. But her jaw literally dropped when she saw my physical frailty.

After about ten minutes of talk, she suddenly hit me with, "How much do you want to live?"

My answer was stunned silence.

"I'll take that to mean you really don't want to survive," she said, challenging me.

Was she right? After all, what did I have to live for? I had endured a lifetime of mental fog and low self-esteem with psychotic interludes. I was living only because my suicide would have crushed my family.

So the first order of the day was to fan the flames of survival. In order to do that, I had to begin creating a life that was fulfilling and rewarding. Eager to learn, I took a little notebook so I could write down her pearls of wisdom. Years of wanting to run and hide had to be met with a new way of thinking.

But, first things first. I had to start eating weight-producing foods.

Caroline found me to be a hard nut to crack. According to all the reading I'd done, psychotic episodes may be triggered by allergy-producing foods in some people. For two years, I'd eaten only salads and fruits. Breads were out because they would likely produce yeast. The naturopath who had nearly killed me told me that anything else could produce a hallucination. With that kind of false advise, that "doctor" helped me develop a real food phobia.

Session after weekly session revolved around my food intake, only ending in frustration for both of us. I couldn't or wouldn't break my dietary anxieties.

Finally, one day she played hardball.

"Barbara, what difference does it make if your diet makes your thinking hazy? You won't have to worry about that if you're dead. If you don't gain weight, you're going to die!" This time she leaned forward and skewered me with her eyes.

With my new-found desire to live, I began slowly to release my food hang-ups. At the nearby health food store, The Natural Way, I purchased whole grain breads, fruit and produce, and bought my meat and fish elsewhere. Sixty pounds rolled on within a year. This new-found health was great!

Sometimes simple works best. Lying on a couch wouldn't have produced the same results as this truly balanced diet did.

Somewhere around the tenth visit, Caroline gave me a list of twenty symptoms associated with prolonged trauma or abuse. I identified with all but three.

The ensuing years of therapy focused on the twin issues of alcoholism and abuse. I had the intense heat of rage inside of me, a white-hot fury that needed to be channeled and neutralized.

Caroline encouraged me to release the anger rather than repressing it as I had in the past. She suggested I write in a journal, talk it out, and beat the stuffing out of all my pillows.

She also sent me to Lenore Schulein, who specializes in anger management.

The walls of her office are padded, so at the peak of anger release, a client can grab a bataka (a small sturdy racket) and physically attack the walls. On my last visit, I broke one of them – and I graduated.

CHAPTER TWENTY-NINE

Painting New Pictures: 1989, Age 46

Unlike the bataka, the technique of reframing or shifting perspective remains one of my favorite coping mechanisms. Using that method, Caroline taught me to symbolically confront my father, thereby reclaiming my power.

As close as I can recall, the first internal dialogue went something like this: "Dad, when you come home drunk nearly every night, I feel so hopeless and actually sick to my stomach. Sometimes I wish you'd plow into a tree and die so I wouldn't have to see you like that ever again, which makes me feel guilty and that cuts into my opinion about myself.

"You've got to get treatment. I'll be there for you, encouraging you."

(Reader: Notice that I was using present tense verbs, even though he'd been dead for thirteen years.)

Even though this conversation took place in my head, I'd begun to discover my inner strength and my voice.

Reframing continues to be a blessing in rewriting the script of my life and of every wrenching event. At Caroline's direction,

I decided to go into each traumatic scene and recast it in a new healthier light.

The giant ant, oh what a horror that was! Yes, that hallucination scared the wits out of me. But the Brown Cow was exciting! During meditation one morning, I focused on that event until the feelings of elation and joy superseded the anxiety I had at that time. The yummy taste of that ice cream was still crystal clear after more than fifty years.

Later that evening, I went to The Natural Way and bought another one. This time it landed in my stomach instead of on the hot sidewalk, and a new energy surged into my being.

What had happened just before I saw my father drunk for the first time? I was having a wonderful time with the family at grandma's house, eating doughnuts and having ice cubes put down my back.

Choice. What a wonderful word.

What were the events before our chilling conversation about my old classmate's child molestation arrest? I remembered taking my nephews to the park for our weekly picnic lunch and long walk. I loved spending time with those sweet little boys. They were and are the light of my life. So I chose to meditate on the pleasure of being with them.

A recent reunion prompted me to apply the same technique to memories about high school. I came home from that event emotionally drained, having relived the feelings of anxiety and isolation that haunted my school days. I decided to reframe those unhappy events, finally remembering one funny event from back then. It involved sneaking into the nuns' living quarters.

Now, in the Catholic tradition of the sixties, any invasion into the cloister could be punishable by excommunication from the Church. When I arrived at the top of the steps of the nuns' house, I met the scariest human being I'd ever laid eyes on. She probably was a sweet little nun, but to me she was Godzilla, especially when she said, "What're you doing here?"

Neither of us knew who the other one was. She had no time to recognize me, and I didn't stick around long enough to know her. Racing back down the steps, I had visions of my parents being informed of my downfall and expulsion from the Church and the school.

Other humorous events occurred to me during that prayer session and gave a whole new vibration to my thoughts about high school. I was in the process of choosing my response to my memories. How empowering it's been to have awareness of options!

Over time, with help from my therapist, my church, and God, my circumstances have lost their power, the victim has left, and the survivor has arrived.

CHAPTER THIRTY

Group Therapy: 1998, Age 55

My time in Caroline's office has provided me with the tools to deal with my challenges and put me in the driver's seat. The first tool was reframing. The next involved five of her women clients who had experienced depression and abuse, including me. At her suggestion, I also participated in a few similar groups before and after this one met. But this one proved to be the most positive for me.

Unfortunately, we only had four sessions. As it turned out, our job commitments made it impossible to continue.

All of us were working through old parental abuse.

At the first meeting, as often happens, I arrived ten minutes late and immediately recognized a long-time friend and her golden retriever support dog. I'd never met the other three women. As soon as I sat down, she handed out the Beck Depression Inventory, which was designed to access our mood levels at that time.

We introduced ourselves by first name only and gave brief rundowns of our life stories. That took the whole hour.

At the second meeting, we settled ourselves into one or another of the overstuffed or straight-backed chairs. Caroline handed out large white poster boards on which we were to draw free-form pictures with colored markers. Our images were to depict our strengths and life interests. Mine had a keyboard, a treble and a bass clef sign, notes, a guitar, and a Bible. The other boards showed a big gentle dog, a typewriter, a steno pad, a ruler, a piece of chalk, and a blackboard. One participant created a striking, highly artistic picture of a rose surrounded by a halo of yellows, oranges, and blues.

These concrete images took us past our emotional garbage and into a positive self-identity.

During the life-board project, two of the members remained silent and self-absorbed. Neither made eye contact with others. Their drawings were tight and sparse. The other members and I were the verbal ones, and our drawings, especially mine, sprawled all over the board. I was pleasantly startled at my active place in the group dynamics. If it weren't for Caroline, I could cheerfully have taken over.

My internal dialogue began with judgment. *Why don't they look up and join in? Barbara, you're looking in the mirror. No wonder my behaviors have bugged others.* And it was scary to realize that I could so easily lapse into that again. I knew I'd come a long way.

At that point, we began to warm up to each other. Caroline had successfully shifted the balance so that we three talkers actually listened to the other two as they began to open up.

When we met for the fourth session, Caroline again handed out the twenty-question test. The result? We all had lower depression and anxiety scores. As we prepared to leave, Caroline offered these words of advice: "Remember, the ball's in your court. You can choose to remain depressed or you can take control of your lives. Observe healthy people and emulate their behaviors."

This became my mantra.

CHAPTER THIRTY-ONE

Observe and Emulate: 2002, Age 59

Observe and emulate – what a powerful belief! As a survivor and conqueror of flat affect, I now sought to move in a more positive direction. I started learning from people who were active participants in the joy of life and became fascinated with nonverbal communication.

A few years after Caroline's magical words, I took part in a Memorial Day peace rally at a local church.

About forty of us listened to a day-long program which included the pastor, several politicians, and a passionate keynote speaker, Abdullah Shariff. He represented a group called Commonway and spoke for over an hour on the very serious topic of global conflict resolution.

After a short break in the fellowship hall, we returned to the sanctuary to meet the wild and crazy musical group called "Joia." They handed each of us a rhythm band instrument ranging from traditional to funky, after which we all paraded out of the church, sashaying the six sidewalk blocks to Carondelet Park.

What a happy group we were and what an exuberant sound we made! Beating on drums – from the giant booming kind, to the little djembe, to dressed-up coffee cans, and some rattling, sassy maracas – we certainly did capture the attention of any and all passersby.

At the park, we settled down at picnic tables to feast on burgers, potato salad, and watermelon. The mood of the group was light and playful. A few drifted off to walk the portable labyrinth and visit various booths set up by civic and church groups.

I had deliberately sat next to the keynote speaker. With his energizing speech still vibrating in my head, I couldn't wait to sound him out on some of his key points, like improved communications between disparate Middle East groups. Unfortunately, he was only interested in his hamburger and chose not to get into a "real" conversation. I was both disappointed and crestfallen. Even as my horizons grew brighter, the flashbacks of rejection caused me pain.

Instead of wallowing, I decided to listen to the conversation styles of my table mates. After the serious tone of the day, they just wanted to have fun. The talking consisted of short comments about the luscious watermelon and homemade brownies. Faces and responses reflected the upbeat mood of the picnic.

I needed to become more in tune with the mood of the conversation of the moment.

Another prime opportunity to build my social skills came from the weekly lunches after services at my home church. By that time, eye contact was okay, but enjoying a lively conversational give and take with both words and facial expressions, remained a challenge. In addition to our shared vocations in teaching and music, we all love a good political discussion. But when I first joined the lunch group in 2002, I still felt socially awkward. Negative comparisons to others interfered with feelings of confidence and positive self-esteem. Aching memories of my music internship and job "failures" continued to dampen my spirits from time to time.

Gradually, after several of Reverend Marigene's sermons on living in the present and letting go of the past, I took the first shaky steps away from my self-defeating thoughts and moved on to the path of wholeness.

At those lunches, I observed that each of us had our own style. One had a fabulous sense of humor, another used hand gestures and smiles, and another sat quietly and actively listened, which showed in her body language. There was no single right way to communicate with others.

Over time, confidence has grown in these lunch situations, and I'm now able to hold my own in the conversations.

Sunday school was another matter altogether. Even after seven monthly sessions of teaching fourth and fifth graders, I was still the typical overwhelmed neophyte. But then I was joined by my assistant teacher, Mary DiMatto, who put her Special School District talents to use. The small functional, but cluttered room quaked with twelve rambunctious kids, one of whom chose to kick a soccer ball around the table.

How could we channel their energy into that day's lesson? Mary, with wisdom born of experience, corralled those children with eye contact, smiles, and personal greetings, addressing those she knew by name, including those she didn't know with honest good cheer. She seemed to sparkle with enthusiasm.

Mary looked around the room and spotted a cracked back-of-the-door mirror that was destined for the dumpster. With an uncanny knack for using whatever was at hand, she turned it into an instrument of teaching the children that what they give out, they will get back. As with life, if they looked into it with anger, they got anger back, and if they looked into it with love, they got love back.

I watched with fascination! So that's how it's done! Involve them by connecting with each and every one and use whatever props are available. I can do that!

So often, it's not the lesson, but how we learn it. God bless observation.

CHAPTER THIRTY-TWO

Songs and Social Skills: June 2005, Age 62

Choir singing offered me another opportunity to work on my social skills and general self-confidence. Monday is choir rehearsal night at the Center for Spiritual Living. It was my first practice with them, and being unfamiliar with their procedures, I sat down absent-mindedly in a random, open chair, which prompted one of the men to quizzically ask, "Has your voice changed?"

"No, I just like to expand my vocal range now and then." Chagrined, I quickly moved out of the bass section to the soprano side.

After loosening up our voices with a few warm-up exercises, choir director Jean Gray led us in several choral selections.

We opened our folders to "Celebrate Life" and began to sing. Unaccustomed to singing with a choir, I soon discovered I needed to reduce my decibel level drastically since this was hardly a solo performance. Me, the woman who had experienced such trouble speaking, was now singing too loudly.

When the choir director asked, "Who wants to take the high note?" I screwed up my courage and volunteered to sing the high G. The first time we got to the end, I took a deep breath, hoped for the best, only to succeed in silence. The second time, a moderate squawk emerged. On the verge of giving up, I tried a third time and came out with a semi-pleasant squeal. The fourth try produced a nice round tone, good, if not operatic.

Just like life, you have to keep trying until you hit the right note. I no longer had to lip-sync as I did in the Fontbonne choir.

For the next few songs, we all sounded quite professional. Our director pushed us to perfection while encouraging lots of fun and fellowship in the process. After forty-five years of silence, I was thoroughly enjoying myself.

I reveled in the camaraderie, only occasionally becoming too exuberant in my efforts to appear vibrant and alive. And I basked in this exciting, new-found social life.

CHAPTER THIRTY-THREE

Trial and Error: 2004, Age 61

Success in overcoming mental health challenges is often about trial and error, setting obtainable goals, and exercising persistence and determination.

We take three steps forward, one back, and another forward. Learning from our errors ensures progress. And along the way, it's healthy to give ourselves permission to make mistakes rather than throwing up our hands and quitting.

When someone takes up a musical instrument, bloopers are made, and mastery occurs in tiny increments. When I decided to take trumpet lessons a few years ago, I brought a few squawks into my house. My daring cat, Blossom, learned to exit the room whenever the trumpet came out. In my futile efforts to sound like Winston Marsalis, I made some painful noises and always later apologized to poor Blossom's ears. After six months of trial and terror, I managed to produce a pretty good version of "Ode to Joy," and my cat relaxed.

Getting on a bike the first time presented similar challenges. Uncle Bud took on the role of teacher. Eager to begin, I grabbed the handle bars and began to pedal while he protectively held onto the seat. As I wobbled back and forth, scared out of my mind, he encouraged me to keep going. So I kept moving my feel rhythmically until I felt the bicycle rolling freely. Bud was standing a half block away! He had let go, and I was riding by myself. Panic set in and down I went, scraping my knee into a bloody pump. With a bandage healing my wound and Aunt Girlie's hugs healing my heart, I was soon back on the bike, riding confidently and accident free. I had to fall before I rode successfully.

Of course, every dance class experience involves trial and error. How many of us have stumbled over our feet trying to imitate Astaire and Rogers? While working at Bethesda as an activity aide, I signed up for tap at a local arts center. My predecessor tap danced to entertain the residents and had a reputation for actively engaging them. Maybe doing likewise would improve my job rating. At each class, we had to warm up with a few basic routines. Try following an eight year old who flits around the room like Shirley Temple! My feet didn't want to do anything in the right order. During the first of our ten sessions, we were taught the basis choreography of "Puttin' On the Ritz." My own routine went like this: do a shuffle beat, fall on the floor, tap one, two, three, and trip over my shoe. Would I never get this down pat? I'm happy to say, I was finally able to conquer it.

We achieve our goals by moving forward in tiny increments. In that way, we can climb the mountains of life one step at a time.

Certainly, I learned to drive "in tiny increments." When I was fifteen, my friend, Rosemary Banayat, put me behind the wheel of her 1962 Dodge. With both of our lives in danger, I took charge and promptly drove over a large bump.

Over the next few years, after tortuous sessions with and ear-splitting screams from my father, I flunked the driving test a grand total of three times. Finally, in my twenties, I took a driver's ed class at Webster Groves High School. The car felt like a war zone. All those gadgets confused me at first. How do I manage the steering wheel, the gas pedal, and the signals? Driving behind Hixson Middle School seemed safe enough, but getting out on the road scared me. Still, I couldn't stay in the parking lot forever. Turning corners, putting on the brake, and checking the rear view mirror can make one feel completely dyslectic. Believe me, I took quite a few lessons and did a lot of practice driving before finally passing the test.

Small steps also helped me overcome my fear of crowds.

A large part of my family time involved participation in the Catholic Church Mass and attending weekly church services, neighborhood rosaries, and meal-time prayers. They all played an important role in our family life.

The Church doesn't look kindly on one missing Sunday services and neither did my family. Over time, I developed a crippling fear of crowds, making attendance a weekly agony. Rather than roasting in Hell, I chose to confront my problems. Wearing a watch with a second hand, I forced myself to sit in the pew for a minimum of sixty seconds and left at the first hint of a panic attack. I was developing a brand new muscle and had to do it slowly. The following week, I stayed a minute longer. Fortunately, my baby steps propelled me steadily forward and I never regressed. It took two years before I could sit through a whole mass. What a hallelujah moment!

Likewise, this book was achievable because I wrote one word, one sentence, and one chapter at a time, determined not to set myself up for failure. Writing it out by hand on a tear-spotted spiral notebook drained me. From time to time, I put it down for a few weeks at a time because the emotional strain was almost unbearable. My friends, Kenneth and Louise Portwine, painstakingly typed it out word for word and returned a two-hundred page, single-spaced manuscript to me. Apparently, major cutting had to be done to my excessively wordy book.

Instead of feeling discouraged, I decided to get to work and finish what I'd started. Awareness of the complexity of this project gave me pause. But putting one foot in front of the other, step by step, made it feel achievable.

Strong determination plays an important role in overcoming fears. Big things don't concern me. I'm bothered by little fears, like going down escalators. It's embarrassing to be with people who hop on those moving stairs while I have to find the elevator. Talk about feeling stupid!

In 2004, when I attended the annual World Piano Cup competition in Cincinnati, I was in the Westin Hotel with one of my students and her family. Once again, as we all approached the escalator, I chose to take the elevator. Since I didn't take the time to explain my situation, they all proceeded up the escalator and lost me in the process. The elevator took a year and forever to show up on the ground floor so by the time I got to the second floor, the whole family was looking for me. I apologized all over myself, admitting my fear of escalators.

This would be the last year of that! I got mad!

I went back to the Four Point Sheraton, where I was staying, and decided to master that darn thing! The following day, I approached it with resolve. I tried unsuccessfully two or three times to go up the escalator.

I finally told myself, *"the hell with it. I'm tired of being different and afraid to do things other don't think twice about.* I took God with me and stormed it with more zeal than the Allies on D-day and up, up, up I went, up to the second floor, the third floor, the fourth floor. I was on a roll. (Ha! - great pun)

Heights have also presented a challenge. Think about going up and down the Statue of Liberty. Those steps are absolutely forbidding. Not wanting to be the odd one out during my high school senior trip to New York, I grudgingly went along with my class, feeling terrified the entire time. *"God help me,"* I thought as I looked down on Manhattan from the top. *"Why can't the whole world be at eye level?"* If going up was Chinese torture, coming back down was worse than water boarding. With about half my class behind me, I somehow lost a shoe about half-way to the ground and had to walk to the next level on one foot. Only sheer grit moved me forward.

CHAPTER THIRTY-FOUR

Mastering Fears: 2008, Age 65

In my own journey to wellness, I've used multiple methods to achieve wholeness.

Patience can be one powerful key to mastering fears. Slow progress is often followed by welcomed achievement. How often have I experienced writer's block, only to persist through my frustration and suddenly be hit with a breakthrough? I sat down to write the first paragraph of this book in 2003 and six years later, I'm seeing completion. Numerous computer breakdowns, printer woes, and tears have blocked progress many times. But patience and perseverance propelled me forward.

Fliers advertising my expertise in music therapy were mailed out in 1995. Two years later, the activities director at a local assisted living center responded by hiring me. Results were not immediate, making it necessary to exercise delayed gratification.

The same applies in the pursuit of learning a major musical work. Beethoven wrote five piano concertos, four of which were, at one time, in my repertoire. Learning Concerto Number One in C Major took an entire year. From the first note forward to the last brilliant chord, I perspired, plodded, persevered, and finally won a local competition with a performance of the first glorious movement. What patience that took!

How does this apply to mastering fears? Let me explain. I know someone who chose to walk the high wire so she could successfully write about the Flying Wallendas. Could I do such a thing? It's not too likely. I don't even like to get up on a chair to change a light bulb!

A few weeks ago, two of the track lights in my music studio burned out, and teaching piano in the dark doesn't work too well. Try reading music, counting, and working on theory pages in a pitch black room!

I had a bit of a conundrum. Either fix the situation or ask the parent of a student to help me out. Although I felt ridiculous, I chose the latter and she had the job done in less than a minute.

Will I live my whole life being unable to perform such a basic task? Truthfully, who cares? Still, there's a certain lack of self-esteem involved in my fear of doing something so simple. So I set about to correct the situation.

I stood on the chair until the first panic attack hit. After stepping down for a few minutes, I tried again. Six attempts later, I was able to stand long enough to begin to feel secure. Then I held the track light until the panic subsided again. Each additional attempt brought greater confidence. Finally, the bulb went into place.

Adopting a different style of inner dialogue can be a potent tool in dealing with panic. Positive self-talk carries a strong healing energy. As a child, I absorbed my father's doomed view of humanity as being lowly creatures subject to God's desire to crush us at will. What a sad, disempowering thought! He no doubt carried this forth from his own upbringing and passed it down to me, an innocent recipient. His teaching became my belief. As an adult, I needed to find a new way to reword this.

So I've adopted a new self-talk vocabulary.

We are children of God, made in His image and likeness, born to be an original blessing. We are reflections of His love, kindness, and respect. Since we are all part of His plan, we possess the ability to bring good into the world.

Scrap the powerless victim image and welcome the magnificence of survival and forward motion of positive changes.

Mental health challenges can bring a tremendous sense of shame and isolation, but well-led group work can help to restore a sense of belonging.

Is a diabetic dumb? Is a cancer patient incompetent? Is a paraplegic mentally impaired? Anxiety disorder is every bit as pathological as any other ailment, and it may require physical and psychological intervention, which includes one-on-one and group counseling sessions. When led by experts, groups can provide valuable, mutual encouragement and acceptance among the participants.

These therapeutic counseling groups come in a variety of settings, including both autonomous, long-term situations run by members, and short-term group therapy sessions facilitated by mental health professionals.

I have experienced excellent results in all types of group settings. Sometimes, traditional open-ended situations (especially those that are member-led support meetings) can degenerate into extended periods of retelling old stories with little opportunity for positive change. I attended one such group for over a year and dropped out because of minimal, if any, progress.

However, the occasional "stuck" group does not negate the purpose and usual effectiveness of such regular gatherings. Those of us who have endured trauma need safe places to identify the sources of our pain. It's healthy to simply be aware that different groups have different kinds of sharing, and it's wise to shop around for one that's a good fit for you.

Professionally facilitated encounters, on the other hand, offer a different approach. Called group therapy rather than support groups, they are managed by a qualified counselor who can guide the members back into productive exchanges if the meetings become too negative.

There is a third category. These are long-term, open-ended assemblies conducted by a professional, as opposed to group members. I've also found this type of setting to be helpful because once again, group energy can be changed by a trained mental health expert if members slip into the victim mode.

Talk with your own counselor or clergyman about which kind would benefit you the most, and then visit more than one before you "settle in."

The Feathered Parade

Once upon a time, several drivers at Garden View Care Center came across seventeen tiny goslings making their way across the parking lot, heading straight for McDonald's.

What a nuisance they were, blocking the way for such a long line of cars.

A few hungry and disgruntled drivers threw their arms up in frustration.

But wait! Something magical seemed to be happening. One little feathered guy was limping.

The other sixteen could have ambled along, leaving him behind. But they chose to adapt to his pace, nudging and encouraging him.

They seemed to be saying, *come on little one, with our help you can make it. You're not alone. We're walking the walk with you.*

The strong helped the injured.

Little gosling didn't feel alone and useless because his companions treated him as healthy and in need of a bit of assistance. Counselors and doctors, ministers and rabbis, friends and family, you are in a position to help those who suffer from depression, psychosis, and anxiety so we don't feel so isolated and lonely.

You are the healthy goslings guiding the impaired.

Thank you . . .

SECTION 2

Mental Disorders & Treatments

Introduction

The current complete list of recognized mental disorders, shown in the *DSM-IV-FR* (Wiley 2004) requires 1,382 pages and weighs 7.1 pounds. Written for use by the mental health community, it's highly detailed and includes both descriptions and treatments.

Since this section of *Recovering from Depression, Anxiety, and Psychosis* is just one brief chapter, you may have guessed that it covers only a few of the more common illnesses and a bare sampling of the possible treatments. For the latter, you'll find both traditional therapies and alternative (or complementary) therapies in the following pages. The chapters will give the reader a sense of the causes and symptoms of a few disorders and an overview of the therapies now in use. With so many treatments available, the odds of being able to help sufferers of mental illness have never been greater.

- Information for the "Mental Disorders" chapter came from the websites of Mayo Clinic, National Institute of Mental Health, Stanford University, National Alliance on Mental Illness, American Psychiatric Association, the U.S. Department of Health and Human Services, and the American Psychological Association. Some information is experimental, learned through personal experience and interviews.

NEVER STOP, BEGIN, OR ADJUST THE DOSAGE OF ANY
MEDICINE, TREATMENT, OR OTHER MEDICAL REGIMEN,
EITHER TRADITIONAL OR ALTERNATIVE,
WITHOUT FIRST CONSULTING YOUR MEDICAL DOCTOR!

KEEP BOTH YOUR MEDICAL DOCTORS AND
ALTERNATIVE PHYSICIANS UPDATED ON ALL
TRADITIONAL AND ALTERNATIVE MEDICATIONS
OR TREATMENTS, INCLUDING HERBALS,
THAT YOU ARE CURRENTLY ON.

CHAPTER ONE

Descriptions of a Few Mental Health Disorders

DEPRESSION

Depression is a serious medical illness affecting fifteen million Americans in any given year. This estimate undoubtedly understates the number of those affected. It can range from situational sadness to major depression and involves both physical and mental well-being. Sufferers cannot snap out of it by using willpower alone, although time can help heal some event-induced depressions.

There's a wide range of types of depression from feeling blue to chronic debilitation, that interfere with daily life.

Major depression, also known as unipolar or clinical depression, is marked by severe insomnia, difficulty concentrating (brain fog), eating disorders (such as bulimia), and an inability to experience pleasure. It can block word recall, logical thought progression, reasoning, and both verbal and written communication.

Most health professionals consider major depression a chronic illness requiring long-term treatment. Although some suffers may have repeated episodes throughout life, others go through only one such experience. Effective treatment and diagnosis can help reduce even severe depression symptoms and can enable most patients to feel better within weeks and be able to return to previously enjoyed daily activities.

A few other kinds of depression are the following:
- Dysthymia is less disabling than major depression, but it still causes disruption in significant areas of life.
- Psychotic Depression involves delusions and hallucinations.
- Postpartum Depression can occur after the birth of a child.
- Seasonal Affective Disorder (SAD) occurs during winter months, when natural sunlight is at a low ebb.
- Bipolar Disorder involves wide mood swings.

ANXIETY DISORDERS

Anxiety disorders include panic disorder, obsessive-compulsive disorder, post traumatic stress disorder (PTSD), phobias, and generalized anxiety disorder.

Descriptions and symptoms are generally as follows:

Panic Disorder is experienced as sudden panic attacks bordering on stark terror. Panic victims may become anxious just anticipating another attack. Symptoms may include the following:
- Heart palpitations
- Shortness of breath
- Losing touch with reality
- Fear of losing their mind and possibly becoming violent

Identifying panic triggers may help victims to rearrange their lives to avoid those hot buttons.

Note: ER physicians often see patients who mistakenly interpret the chest pain and tightness as a heart attack, the fear of which only adds to the panic.

Obsessive Compulsive Disorder (OCD) manifests as incessant and irrational repetition of otherwise normal actions. The unrelenting, pointless urges or rituals can prevent OCD patients from living normal lives. These repeated behaviors may involve the following:
- Locking doors
- Washing hands
- Counting, i.e., ceiling tiles, bricks, or parking meters
- Cleaning and rearranging objects, etc.

Post Traumatic Stress Disorder (PTSD) can strike after a severe traumatic event, either physical or emotional. Frequently diagnosed in war veterans who may relive the stress of intense battle, it's also seen in survivors of natural disasters like hurricane Katrina, as a result of childhood abuse, or from terrifying and life-threatening situations. It's often devastating, resulting in nightmares, flashbacks and crippling depression, and insomnia, and may not manifest until weeks or months after the triggering event.

Healthy coping mechanisms, plus a strong support system can help in the management process. Sometimes, however, PTSD can cause serious life interruptions.

Symptoms usually fall into one of these types:
- Intrusive Memories – Reliving the trauma over and over for minutes and sometimes even days at a time
- Spontaneous flashbacks
- Debilitating nightmares about the original event
- Avoidance Symptoms – Staying away from events or places that are reminders of the trauma
- Numbing out physically and emotionally
- Depression
- Loss of one's ability to take pleasure in previously enjoyed activities
- Hyperarousal – High startle reflex, becoming easily angered or experience extreme rage
- Inappropriate guilt or shame
- Crippling insomnia

- Psychotic hallucinations
- Self-Destructive Behavior – Including alcoholism, cutting, and eating disorders among others

Phobias are characterized by irrational, intense fear of situations or objects. The disabling reactions can range from moderate anxiety to extreme physical symptoms.

According to the National Institute of Mental Health (NIMH), over 19 million adults in the U.S. experience specific phobias with twice as many women as men so affected. Avoidance of the trigger often keeps the fears at bay. However, if that interferes with normal activities, treatment from a mental health professional may be sought. Claustrophobia (fear of enclosed places), arachnophobia (fear of spiders), acrophobia (fear of heights), fear of flying, dogs, snakes, storms, tunnels, and bridges are among the more common phobias.

Many also suffer from social phobia and fear of public speaking, both of which involve an intense fear of being scrutinized, ridiculed, and harshly judged.

Physical symptoms of phobic reactions may include the following:
- Heart palpitations
- Tightness in the chest
- Shortness of breath
- Upset stomach
- Trembling
- Light-headedness
- Uncontrollable sweating
- Difficulty making eye contact

Generalized Anxiety Disorder (GAD). Occasional anxious feelings are normal. On-going, relentless anxiety, which interferes with every-day life situations and relationships, may indicate the presence of Generalized Anxiety Disorder, which commonly occurs in conjunction with major depression.

People suffering from GAD experience excessive worry over everyday problems for at least six months. Normal challenges become enormous problems. It interferes with daily routines and relationships and makes enjoying life difficult. Symptoms may include the following:

- High startle reflex
- Concentration difficulties
- Insomnia
- Headaches
- Muscle tension and pains
- Problems with swallowing
- Shaking or twitching
- Irritability
- Nausea
- Frequent urination
- Breathlessness

DISSOCIATIVE DISORDERS

As with many forms of mental illness, dissociative disorder symptoms can range from amnesia to alternate (or multiple) personalities in self-protective reaction to traumatic or acutely painful memories. When such events occur, especially in childhood, the mind may cope by stepping away from the situation mentally. Depending on the type of dissociative disorder, symptoms may include the following:

- Loss of memory about certain times, places, and people (amnesia);
- A blurred sense of personal identity;
- A sense of being detached or separate from one's self (depersonalization);
- A distorted sense of one's surroundings (derealization).

Sufferers often experience other mental health problems as well, such as depression, anxiety, and post-traumatic stress disorder. The four major types of this disorder are as follows.

Dissociative Identity Disorder. Formerly called Multiple Personality Disorder, this involves an individual having two or more distinct, alternative personalities. The different personalities can have strikingly different styles, voices, physical traits (needs eyeglasses or not), and be either male or female. One or more of the individual personalities may not know of the existence of the other(s).

Dissociative Fugue. Onset is often sudden and results from a single traumatic event. The sufferer abruptly leaves his or her home, adopts a partial or completely new identity, and goes on a journey, which can last from hours to months. The experience usually ends spontaneously and does not recur.

Depersonalization Disorder. This disorder is primarily distinguished by a feeling of being separate from one's mind and body, simply going through the motions of living. The sense of being out of touch and out of control creates a feeling of being "spaced out," and may become so severe that the outside world seems distorted.

SCHIZOPHRENIA

This psychotic disorder, lasting at least six months, is characterized by two or more of the following: delusions, hallucinations, severe disorganization, catatonic behavior, and inappropriate language. Subtypes include the following:
- Paranoid Type – delusions and hallucinations of being persecuted;
- Disorganized Type – exhibits disorganized speech or regressive behavior, flat affect or social withdrawal;
- Catatonic Type – severely reduced or amplified speech or behavior;
- Undifferentiated Type – may have delusions, hallucinations, and flat affect, but does not fit the criteria of any specific type of schizophrenia;
- Residual Type – patients have experienced one or more acute schizophrenic bouts, but not exhibit strong, specific, symptoms at present, indicating the disorder has not been completely resolved.

SCHIZOPHRENIA-LIKE DISORDERS

Schizophreniform Disorder. With this disorder, sufferers exhibit symptoms of schizophrenia, but completely recover, indicating that the original cause has not yet been discovered.

Schizoaffective Disorders. Schizoaffectives display some of the characteristics of schizophrenics, but to a lesser degree and involve both mood disorder and psychosis.

Brief Psychotic Episode. Characterized by a single, isolated episode lasting for more than one day, but less than a month.

OTHER PSYCHOTIC DISORDERS

Delusional Psychosis. Nonbizarre symptoms occur for at least a month, but without other symptoms of schizophrenia.

Shared Psychotic Episode. An episode shared with someone else who suffers the same delusions.

Psychotic Disorder Due to Medical Condition. Psychosis due to epilepsy, medications for Parkinson's, head trauma, or stroke.

Psychotic Disorder Not Otherwise Specified. Symptoms do not fit the above definitions.

Substance Abuse Psychosis. Psychosis related to drug abuse.

This chapter is obviously just a bare sampling of mental illness. But I hope the above information helps my readers to better understand the causes, feelings, and specific problems of these disabilities.

CHAPTER TWO

Traditional Medical Treatments

Traditional health care professionals, including psychiatrists, medical doctors, psychologists, and social workers, talk at length with the patient and perhaps administer tests to determine the appropriate treatment for that person.

Only psychiatrists and medical doctors can legally write prescriptions for drugs, which primarily fall into one of these categories:

- SSRIs – (selective serotonin reuptake inhibitors, including Prozac, Zoloft, and Praxil)
- SNRIs – (serotonin and norepinephrine reuptake inhibitors, including Effexor and Cymbalta)
- MAOs – (monoamine oxidase inhibitors, including Nardil and Marplan)
- Tricyclic antidepressants – (including Aventyl and Sinequan)
- Beta Blockers – (including Lopressor and Inderal)
- Other medications, like lithium, are less commonly required

Most of these drugs come in various strengths and may be combined for a synergistic effect. Not all drugs work equally well for all patients, and the doctor may need to reduce or increase dosage or prescribe a different medication if the first or second one either isn't effective or produces ongoing, unacceptable side effects.

Patients can become discouraged when adjustments have to be made either to increase effectiveness or alleviate ongoing side effects, but supportive family and friends can help them through those times with love and understanding.

It's vital that the patient check in with the prescribing doctor on a regular basis to be sure that their current regimen is still fully effective and doesn't need adjustment. Occasionally, the drug or dosage may need to be changed.

CHAPTER THREE

Counseling

Most health care providers recommend counseling or psychotherapy either in addition to or instead of medications. Psychologists and social workers specialize in counseling through talk therapy, and some psychiatrists offer it in addition to medications.

The scars of false guilts, erroneous parental messages, and the ongoing pain of past emotional traumas often interfere with living a healthy fulfilling life and can be very difficult to uncover. A professional therapist will work with the client to explore and deal with the old emotional pains.

Positive interactive chemistry between client and counselor is essential to healing. Therapists themselves recommend that clients get a list of recommendations, then call and talk to prospective therapists to find the best fit. (Some people prefer to counsel with their pastor, rabbi, or other spiritual leader.)

Short-Term Counseling

In short-term counseling, a licensed professional assesses the client's situation and determines an effective course of therapy. The length of therapy, sadly, is set by insurance companies unless the client chooses to pay for additional sessions out-of-pocket. (Check with your therapist to see if she offers a cash payment discount.)

The exceptions may be situational anxiety or depression, such as grief or some phobias, in which only that single distressing factor will be addressed.

But discovering and working through a troubled emotional history seldom fits into six tidy counseling sessions no matter what the insurance company offers!

Long-Term Counseling

When the therapist needs to explore an entire lifetime or period of the client's life, ongoing counseling will usually be required, and neither therapist nor client can realistically set a completion date for the sessions. (For financial reasons, the client may need to space the sessions farther apart or even take a short break, whereas an acute emotional crisis may call for more frequent sessions.) The function of counseling is to help clients trace their emotional baggage to the origin of their dysfunction. Those negative hot buttons had to come from somewhere.

Group Work

Group work may be recommended in addition to individual sessions. Chapters Thirty-One and Thirty-Four describe the various types and benefits of group work.

CHAPTER FOUR

Complementary (Alternative) Therapies

In addition to traditional medication and counseling treatments, many choose complementary therapies to use with or instead of standard medications. Be very wary of the alternative practitioner who claims to cure major psychotic disorders. Rather, the treatments seek to alleviate symptoms, such as insomnia, anxiety, and depression, which improves overall health and allows the body to heal itself.

Chiropractic and Mental Health

Chiropractic is an alternative therapy recognizing the basic health of the patient and the body's own ability to heal from emotional stress and trauma, and physical and mental stress. It is concerned with the relationship between the nervous system, efferent neurons and afferent neurons, the spinal column, and the entire nervous system. All of the body's organs and tissues are connected to the spinal column, which is protected by the vertebrae. The theory is that the misalignment of the spinal column effects related portions of the body and causes pain, disease, and musculoskeletal abnormalities.

Although there are strict certification standards for chiropractic practice, individual chiropractors often include various other treatments, including acupuncture, kinesiology, and homeopathy in their practice.

Chiropractic may particularly benefit patients who have nervous system problems including depression, schizophrenia, headaches, hearing and ear disorders, sleep disorders, vision disorders, and emotional disturbances.

Naturopathy

Naturopathic doctors use a variety of natural ways of treating and preventing illness and disease in the body, including exercise, lifestyle change, diet, and other therapies in their treatment of the whole person. Like other complementary and alternative treatments, naturopathy does not address specific mental health issues, but rather seeks to raise the patient's health level, with the possibility of relieving or easing symptoms of mental illness.

The basic principles of naturopathy are: first, do no harm; use natural remedies; find the cause; treat the whole person; and, act as the patient's teacher. They employ low-risk methods and healing compounds, including herbal extracts, dietary supplements, and homeopathy.

Look for a licensed naturopathic physician. Upon graduating from a four-year naturopathic medical school, he or she must pass through professional board exams to be licensed as a primary care, general practice physician.

Are herbs safe? All herbs are natural, but they're not all safe. Some plants are extremely toxic or may have negative interactions with standard medications. What's safe for one person isn't necessarily okay for another.

It's important that your naturopathic physician be well grounded in the indications and effects of each herb, and it's best to use only registered practitioners. If prescribed by a qualified naturopath, herbs should be safe if all current traditional medications have been mentioned, and if they are taken in the prescribed dose.

Although there are only a few studies on the effectiveness of naturopathy, there is evidence that anxiety and depression might be alleviated through naturopathic methods.

Warning: It's wise to consult with your primary care physician concerning any herbs taken as a part of naturopathic care because some herbs can interact negatively with traditional medications.

The same is true of homeopathy. The effectiveness of homeopathic medications depends on individual, physiology and constitution. An appropriate dose for one patient may not work for someone else.

Homeopathy

In the 1700s, the brilliant German medical doctor Samuel Hahnemann, developed this therapy based on the principle of similars (like cures like). Homeopathy is designed to stimulate the body's own healing abilities by giving very small doses of extremely dilute substances.

There are homeopathic remedies specifically targeted for mental health issues, and the treatments may help some people with schizophrenia, obsessive compulsive disorder, depression, anxiety, phobias, attention-deficit disorder, and grief. But it's rare that psychotic disorders like the first two will be significantly helped.

Similar to medical approaches to severe mental illness, homeopathic treatments involve a long-term commitment. There are no easy fixes. The homeopathic regimen is geared toward individual needs. A particular remedy may work for one person, but not for someone else. Treatment is given in line with each patient's temperament and personality.

Unlike traditional medicines, clinical research of homeopathic remedies is preliminary. Because individualized responses to homeopathic treatments can vary widely, researchers have yet to develop accurate clinical testing methods. It's a work in progress.

According to the U.S. Department of Health and Human Services, complementary mental health care can also include diet and nutrition, expressive sensory therapies, cultural healing practices, massage, biofeedback, and healing arts from non-Western cultures among others. Many of these can be effective in maintaining mental health as well as easing mental illnesses.

Acupuncture, Ayurvedic medicine, Yoga, Reike, Healing Touch, and Native American practices have been found to be effective in stress reduction. Some of those are meant to improve or correct imbalances within the body and mind, thereby fostering the overall well-being of the patient. Art, dance or movement, and music therapy are examples of expressive therapies.

AUTHOR'S EPILOGUE

I leave you, dear reader, with these final, loving insights about my mother and father.

Honoring My Father
Edward Altman

When I conjure up images of Edward Altman, I can say he went a few steps higher in consciousness and responsibility than my Grandfather Altman. I can't begin to repeat the horrors Dad experienced at the hands of his father. They were far more horrific than the sequence of events my father passed on.

He was a man of extraordinary intelligence, which was largely left unfulfilled. Having only a fourth grade education, he had to start work at a young age to help with family finances.

His fine mental capabilities surfaced in the least likely situation. I used to watch him play Pinochle with my uncles and grandfather. Dad would always be stone drunk and still be able to remember every single card played, who had played what, and who held the remaining cards. He could do this by the second or third round of play. He had perfect memory recall. I'm sure his IQ was extremely high. What a mind! And how it was wasted!

He was absolutely the most detail-oriented person I've ever known. He had a nightly ritual of standing by his dresser drawer and counting every penny in his wallet. Again, he did this in a drunken stupor. Having a thousand dollars in his wallet gave him the self-esteem he lacked. If he was off by 25 cents, my mother and I would cringe until he found it. I would occasionally steal a quarter just for revenge. This is how I expressed anger about his drinking.

And he had the most beautiful handwriting. During his four brief years of education, he was taught the fine art of calligraphy. Only a precocious child could have mastered this. With the proper education and motivation, he could have excelled at almost anything. Unfortunately, demon rum had control over him.

Approximately six months before my father died, the whole family, led by my brother, prayed with him and led him to Christ. He began to cry, asking why he was sobbing if he was so happy.

He had never felt so loved.

Honoring My Mother
Laura Otillia Tritz Altman

What a feisty little bundle of energy, sweetness, and love. Born in Saskatchewan, Canada to nomadic, poverty-stricken farmers, she learned how to appreciate the small things at an early age. She often talked about the joy of getting an orange or a catalog-bought doll at Christmas. They didn't have many worldly goods, but they did have a lot of love.

Her early life was marked by frequent moves and exposure to the cruel whims of nature. While in Texas, she and her twin sister once awakened to the presence of rattlers in their crib. My grandmother lured the snakes away with warm milk.

My grandfather built an outside shelter for protection from the ever-present Texas tornadoes. During one of these horrific storms, the frightened family collected whatever food they could grab and waited out the storm in the shelter, not knowing whether their little home would survive.

Mom had her unique way of showing her love. It was called food. The kitchen was her room, the cook's dynasty. Christmas dinners were on the planning table starting in October. Whether we wanted it or not, we had to eat under the pain of eternal damnation. Rejecting her food was to reject her. She was our Marie from "Everybody Loves Raymond." And what a feast we would have! Our tiny table could barely contain the turkey, ham, pot roast, vegetables, baked potatoes, mustard, and a hundred other items.

Not gifted academically, she had a whole boatload of social intelligence. In her later years, she confessed to being envious of me because I had a college education. I wanted her ability to win friends and influence people. Her smile alone brightened the days of those she knew.

Always devoted to God and the Catholic Church, she held some sort of office in her fifty-plus club at Annunciation Parish in Webster Groves.

To her dying day, she never lost that radiance.

I can see her running some sort of group in heaven.

God bless Laura Otillia Tritz Altman.

APPENDIX A

Recommended Readings

Beattie, Melody. *Codependent No More*. New York: HarperCollins, 1987.

Collins, Judy. *Sanity and Grace*. New York: Penguin Group, 2003.

Donovan, Charles, III. *Out of the Black Hole*. U.E. Williams Publishers, 2006.

Knowles, Jeffrey J. *What of the Night*. Scottdale, Pennsylvania: Harold Press, Waterloo, 1993.

Melody, Pia, and Andrea Wells Miller. *Breaking Free*. San Francisco: HarperCollins, 1989.

Merryman, Rachael. *Broken Promises, Mended Dream*. Little Brown and Company, 1984.

Mooney, Al A., M.D.; Arlene Eisenberg; and Howard Eisenberg. *The Recovery Book*. New York: Workman Publishing, 1992.

Papalos, Demitri, and Janice Demitri. *Darkness Visible*. New York: HarperCollins, 1903.

Teitelbaum, Jacob, M.D. *From Fatigued to Fantastic*. Penguin Group, 2007.

For more information, visit Barbara's website at http://www.depression to recovery.com.

APPENDIX B

Living the Joy–Filled Life: Affirmations

In the past, I've wasted an abundance of energy toward a negative world view. In the present, I'm consistently redirecting my thoughts in a positive direction. I have a set of affirmations I use as aids in shifting my thinking. I enjoy life to the fullest.

I was born to be happy. Suffering becomes joy, rage evolves into forgiveness, abuse becomes respect, and depression becomes happiness.

1. **I embrace forgiveness.** I'm setting myself up for misery if I choose to pitch a tent around anger and resentment.

2. **I don't blame or fault anyone.** Finding fault with others produces soul death. Making my father the master villain castrates my spirit.

3. **The past is over and done. I can't change it. I can only reinvent my response to it.** I can't change the reality of my mental illness, but I can change my perspective. I want to use my voice to bring hope to those afflicted as I have been. That's the purpose I see in my life.

4. **Each experience is an opportunity.** "Failures" can become learning experiences. Losing that internship became one of my life's deepest blessings. It gave me the opportunity to choose to implement major positive changes.

5. **I trust the process of life. I live knowing I'm safe.** Leaping out of the victim mentality spawns growth. I move forward with purpose.

6. **Love surrounds and protects me.** Love is the antidote for fear and apprehension. In fact, I don't even like those words. I only give them space because they're real, but I refuse to give them power. Love begets confidence.

7. **I care for and approve of myself. I speak up for myself. I claim my power.** This hasn't been easy for me. By nature, I'd rather sit back and accept whatever comes my way. It's been my pattern to let others pummel and batter me with no boundaries set on unacceptable behaviors. Admittedly, this is a work in progress.

8. **I'm constantly rewriting my life.** Yesterday's news is in the morgue. I can allow it to murder me or I can release it through forgiveness. I choose the latter.

9. **The victim role is gone.** Out flies the victim. Here comes the survivor.

10. **I see my parents as tiny children who need love. I forgive them and I set them free.** Both of them had challenges growing up, particularly my father. I've looked upon his pain, wept his tears, and felt his anguish. I'll never condone his actions, but I forgive him.

11. **I'm worth loving. I'm worthy of being prosperous. I don't have to earn affection.** I do not need to be fixed. In my spirit I am whole and complete. My behaviors are becoming reflective of God's affection and concern for all of his creation.

Summary

There they are – the big eleven: love of life; forgiveness; the absence of blame; the past is over; every experience is an opportunity; I can trust life; love surrounds and protects me; I care for and approve of myself; I'm constantly rewriting my life; the victim role is gone; I see my parents as tiny children who need love, I forgive them and set them free; and, I'm worth loving, and everyone loves me.

In terms of mental health, I've had four challenges: psychosis, anxiety disorder, depression, and anorexia. They've been met with eleven spiritual solutions. Those odds are unsurpassable.

APPENDIX C

Improving My Health

Removing the Heavy Metals (Aluminum and Mercury)

Controversy abounds over mercury toxicity.

I really don't know if my mercury dental fillings contributed to the development of my psychosis. Theoretically, one person can have a whole mouthful of mercury amalgams and remain symptom-free for life while someone else may have problems with it.

I wasn't willing to take any chances.

In 1999, I made the decision to have all of my amalgams removed. After interviewing three dentists, I set up an appointment with Dr. Michael G. Rehme and proceeded to have them replaced by materials that are chemically compatible with my system.

The process of removal took three visits to complete. Since the age of fifteen, I'd had a persistent feeling of tension in the head and neck. I had frequent spells of a low-grade achy feeling in my temples, lower jaw, and occipital areas. While it didn't kill me with discomfort, the pain was present 24/7. When the last filling came out, the relief was palpable.

I wonder how often valid symptoms are blown off as psychosomatic or how often the sick are treated as hypochondriacs.

Doctors, please take heed and listen to your patients.

In my own search for health, I've implemented a routine that reduces aluminum and mercury in my system. I have a physician who monitors my level of heavy metals and provides sodium dimercaptopropane sulfonate (DMPS) treatments, which are designed to pull them out.

Will this type of treatment help others with mental illness?

I don't know.

My Rules for Healthy Living

The first edict for healthy living is, "Live life with a sense of balance." I've adapted a health-promoting diet that I follow about ninety-five percent of the time, giving myself occasional permission to digress. Sugar bingeing may have played a large part in the development of my psychosis. At the same time, I won't be likely to have a psychotic event if I occasionally have one tiny piece of chocolate. The operative word is "occasionally."

I never use cookware that contains any kind of metals. Even stainless steel contains nickel, which is toxic to the system. I only use glass and Pyrex. I use plastic utensils, not aluminum utensils, unless I'm in a restaurant.

My dietary routine includes plenty of green and yellow foods, meaning a great variety of vegetables with small amounts of protein, an amount about the size of my palm.

Briefly, the don'ts are sugar, yeast, corn, alcohol, peanuts, ice cream, dairy, and soy. All of the above contribute to the overgrowth of yeast, mold, and fungus in the body.

For years, I had symptoms of systemic candida. I despaired of ever overcoming problems with yeast infections. I was telling a friend about this, when she informed me of a routine designed to eradicate this pesky problem.

Dr. Bruce McFarland of Radiance International has a wonderful yeast-eliminating program. It's a seven-stage discipline that takes about nine months to complete.

After more than twenty-five years of persistent infections, I have finally gotten rid of it.

Detox Programs

The same friend recommended someone who specializes in a homeopathic program designed to detoxify each major organ in the body. He also has expertise in neurological problems associated with emotional, physical, and mental challenges and with imbalances in the seven chakra systems.

I've had the privilege of being in his care for the past six years, and I'm now completing his regimen. After about two years of frequent visits, he approached me with the basics and I was immediately interested, especially in the brain detox, which I undertook with enthusiasm.

"Barbara, I think this protocol would be useful for you," he said. "I'll test you to determine which parts of it you need to use."

"Will I experience any reactions?"

"The intensity of symptoms varies from patient to patient. There's no way to determine how anyone will react. Some patients sail through the process with few problems while others are symptomatic. If you do have challenges, they won't be as intense as the original situation."

He was correct. The side effects didn't supersede the horror of those hallucinations and anxiety attacks.

I fell into the latter category of those who had blinding symptoms. With each part of the detox, I had my fair share of headaches, sore throats, backaches, fevers, and fatigue. Being aware of the benefits, I didn't mind going through this process.

Each phase lasted anywhere from seven to ten days to six months, with the brain and thyroid phase being the longest in duration. During each process, I'd wonder just why I was doing this. One can only endure so many headaches or take so much aspirin. However when each segment was completed, I'd go into his office, eager to begin the next step. I was marching toward healing my brain, and I was set to go on to greater physical well-being.

Oh, what torture I endured! Stomachaches and vomiting became routine.

That day came at last. I started on the detox, which took about six months, during which time I had daily headaches, dizziness, problems with balance and coordination, and overall weakness.

I'd classify my response to this protocol as within the range of severe. Occasionally, I'd wake up screaming from wrenching pains in my head. I'd have to take about five aspirins to relieve the discomfort.

About twenty years prior, I'd had a bone marrow test done, showing only twenty-five percent production of red and white cells and platelets. Ever since my teen years, I've had chronic fatigue problems. Part of the detox routine involved clearing out the bone marrow infection. This was excruciating in terms of pain, fatigue, and God-awful headaches.

This program isn't for the faint of heart. My body reacted strongly and produced temporary side effects that would've scared me half to death had I not known what to expect.

I endured it, anticipating health. The effort, expense, and symptoms remain valuable and have significantly improved the quality of my life and my mind.

It's been difficult to go through this, but the benefits have been astounding. I'd do it all again in a minute.

Part of my treatment has included structural work on my spine, a dietary regimen, and a process called cortical integration, which was started about five years ago, prior to going through the detox process.

I've always had excellent fine motor, but poor gross motor coordination. The cortical integration treatments are designed to integrate both hemispheres of the brain, increasing both coordination and ability to concentrate.

Through the next four years, I would show a repeated need for treatments. Thinking I was regressing, I asked my doctor why this had to be done so frequently.

"It's not a matter of experiencing a return to symptoms," he said. "Instead, each treatment builds the connection between the left and right hemispheres. The results will be cumulative."

Looking back at the past five years of combined cortical integration and detox treatments, I stand amazed at the relief I've experienced.

I can laugh, my presence no longer puts people into a state of terminal boredom, and I am totally free of severe dissociative disorder with no fear of ever becoming psychotic again.

Will detox and cortical integration help others with mental illness?

I don't know. I can make no promises.

A Call from God

Over the last ten years, I've had periodic problems with sleep. When my Aunt Girlie became ill in 1999, we knew she had to have help and could no longer live alone. I had been expecting this, but it still hit me with some sudden decisions. When she was hospitalized with pneumonia, I had one week to make plans for her. Should she stay in her home with help from an agency or should she go to assisted living? The poor dear wanted with all her heart to stay in her home. But I worried about bringing in strangers to care for her. That entire week I got about four hours of sleep a night, staying awake and weighing the pros and cons over and over and over.

The sleep issues persisted for about three months until I witnessed her amazing adjustment to her new surroundings at Tesson Heights Retirement Center.

For the next six years, I was back on a good sleep routine. At that time, I was visiting her five to six time a week and dealing with the pressures involved in being her Durable Power of Attorney over health care. In 2006 sleep became a problem again. There were incredible pressures involved over making decisions about her care. With the support of my counselor, I was advised to visit her only two or three times a week. This took care of the insomnia.

Aunt Girlie died in June of 2007. With the help of counselors, church, and friends, I was able to grieve deeply and to take it pretty much I stride.

So when the sleep issue arrived again in 2008, I couldn't figure out what was going on. Again, with the advice of counselors, I decided to hand over the research involved in the second part of this book to my book coach. Looking up information is anathema to me. I'd much rather write freestyle. This temporarily resolved the problem.

But it reoccurred with a vengeance. This time, I would have periodic nights of no sleep at all.

I then consulted my primary care physician, Dr. Christian Wessling, at Webster Family Physicians and was advised to take a neurotransmitter test, which showed very low levels of serotonin and norepinephrine.

I tried to comfort myself, saying that we need less sleep as we age. But I couldn't tolerate the fatigue; I became completely despondent. Finally, during one of my sleepless nights, I cried out to God at 1:00 a.m., 2:00 a.m., 3:00 a.m. until the dawn broke without one ounce of slumber.

"God, if this is to be how my life will be from now on . . ." I felt so hopeless.

The next day at 6:00 p.m., my dear chiropractor friend from Chicago, Dr. Madelein Permutt, called me saying, "Barbara, how are you? I've been thinking about you all day." She asked if I still felt spacey. I told her that I'm no longer dissociated, but concentration is still an issue for me. I also told her about the neurotransmitter test results. She advised getting an Iodine Loading test to determine levels of iodine in my system. I was also placed0 on a comprehensive vitamin, amino acid, and iodine routine designed to improve levels of neurotransmitters in my brain.

Within two weeks, my sleep had improved, and within one month it was completely restored. I no longer fear sleepless nights.

She later told me that she felt an urgency before she called me. She knew even after twelve years of no contact with me that I was in serious straits.

My sleep is back, my mood is improved, and my life has been restored. My mission to impart hope to my readers for healing from depression has been "reflamed."

Dear readers, please check with your internist or your therapist before trying the detox or other approaches I've mentioned. Some are not for the faint of heart, and there are no guarantees.

I know the pain of mental illness, and I bless all those who devote their lives to helping us.

Praise God.

God bless all who have been mentally ill. My prayers are with you.

Made in the USA
Charleston, SC
08 May 2013